Applying Concepts for

Healthy Living

Applying Concepts for

Healthy Living

A Critical-Thinking Workbook

FIFTH EDITION

Sandra Alters, PhD
Wendy Schiff, MS, RD

JONES AND BARTLETT PUBLISHERS
Sudbury, Massachusetts
BOSTON   TORONTO   LONDON   SINGAPORE

World Headquarters
Jones and Bartlett Publishers
40 Tall Pine Drive
Sudbury, MA 01776
978-443-5000
info@jbpub.com
www.jbpub.com

Jones and Bartlett Publishers Canada
6339 Ormindale Way
Mississauga, Ontario L5V 1J2
Canada

Jones and Bartlett Publishers International
Barb House, Barb Mews
London W6 7PA
United Kingdom

Jones and Bartlett's books and products are available through most bookstores and online booksellers. To contact Jones and Bartlett Publishers directly, call 800-832-0034, fax 978-443-8000, or visit our website, www.jbpub.com.

Substantial discounts on bulk quantities of Jones and Bartlett's publications are available to corporations, professional associations, and other qualified organizations. For details and specific discount information, contact the special sales department at Jones and Bartlett via the above contact information or send an email to specialsales@jbpub.com.

Production Credits
Acquisitions Editor: Jacqueline Ann Geraci
Associate Editor: Amy L. Flagg
Production Manager: Julie Champagne Bolduc
Production Assistant: Jessica Steele Newfell
Marketing Manager: Jessica Faucher
Manufacturing Buyer: Therese Connell
Composition: Publishers' Design and Production Services, Inc.
Cover Design: Kate Ternullo and Kristin E. Ohlin
Cover Image: © Martin Ruegner/Radius Images/Masterfile
Printing and Binding: Courier Stoughton
Cover Printing: Courier Stoughton

ISBN 978-0-7637-5755-7

6048

Printed in the United States of America

12 11 10 09 08   10 9 8 7 6 5 4 3 2 1

Contents

Chapter 9

Chapter 10

Chapter 11

Chapter 12

Chapter 13

Chapter 14

Chapter 15

Chapter 16

Chapter 1

SELF-ASSESSMENT 1 Healthstyle

This self-test, which is a modified version of one developed by the U.S. Public Health Service, assesses several health-related behaviors. Although these behaviors apply to most individuals, pregnant women and people with chronic health concerns should follow the advice of their physicians. Answer each of the following questions by circling the number of the response that applies best to you. Add the number of points under each health-related behavior category to obtain a score for that category. Use the scoring guide at the end of the test to determine the level of risk you are incurring by your health-related behavior.

Tobacco, Alcohol, and Other Drugs

If you have never used tobacco products, enter a score of 10 for this section, and skip questions 1 and 2.

	Almost Always	Sometimes	Almost Never
1. I avoid using tobacco products.	(2)	1	0
2. I smoke only low-tar cigarettes.	2	1	(0)

Smoking Score: _2_

	Almost Always	Sometimes	Almost Never
3. I avoid drinking alcoholic beverages, or I drink no more than one or two drinks a day.	(2)	1	0
4. I avoid using alcohol or other drugs (especially illegal drugs) as a way of handling stressful situations or problems in my life.	(2)	1	0
5. I avoid driving while under the influence of alcohol and other drugs.	(2)	1	0
6. I am careful not to drink alcohol when taking certain pain medications or when pregnant.	(2)	1	0
7. I read and follow the label directions when using prescribed and over-the-counter drugs.	(2)	1	0

Alcohol and Other Drugs Score: _10_

Eating Habits

	Almost Always	Sometimes	Almost Never
8. I eat a variety of foods each day, including fruits and vegetables, whole-grain products, lean meats, low-fat dairy products, seeds, nuts, and dry beans.	(3)	1	0
9. I limit the amount of fat that I eat, especially animal fats such as cream, butter, cheese, and fatty meats.	3	1	(0)
10. I limit the amount of salt that I eat, by avoiding salty foods and not using salt at the table.	(2)	1	0
11. I avoid eating too much sugar, by eating few sweet snacks and sugary soft drinks.	2	(1)	0

Eating Habits Score: _6_

Exercise/Fitness

	Almost Always	Sometimes	Almost Never
12. I maintain a body weight that is reasonable for my height.	3	(1)	o
13. I do vigorous exercise (for example, running, swimming, or brisk walking) for at least 30 minutes at least three times a week.	3	1	(o)
14. I do exercises to enhance my muscle tone and flexibility (for example, yoga or calisthenics) for 15 to 30 minutes at least three times a week.	2	1	(o)
15. I use part of my leisure time participating in individual, family, or team activities that increase my level of physical fitness (for example, gardening, bowling, or golf).	(2)	1	o

Exercise/Fitness Score: _3_

Stress Management

	Almost Always	Sometimes	Almost Never
16. I take time every day to relax.	2	(1)	o
17. I find it easy to express my feelings.	2	(1)	o
18. I recognize and prepare for events or situations that are likely to be stressful.	2	(1)	o
19. I have close friends, relatives, or others to whom I can talk about personal matters and contact for help when needed.	2	(1)	o
20. I participate in hobbies that I enjoy or group activities such as religious or community organizations.	2	(1)	o

Stress Management Score: _5_

Safety

	Almost Always	Sometimes	Almost Never
21. I wear a seat belt while riding in a motor vehicle.	(2)	1	o
22. I obey traffic rules and speed limits while driving.	(2)	1	o
23. I have a working smoke detector in my home.	(2)	1	o
24. I am careful when using potentially harmful products or substances, such as household cleaners, poisons, and electrical devices.	2	(1)	o
25. I avoid smoking in bed.	(2)	1	o

Safety Score: _9_

What Your Scores Mean

Scores of 9 or 10 for each section: Excellent! Your responses show that you are aware of the importance of this area to your health, and that you are practicing good health-related habits. As long as you continue to do so, this area of health should not pose a risk.

Scores of 6 to 8 for each section: Your health practices in this area are good, but there is room for improvement. Look at the items that you answered with "Sometimes" or "Almost Never." What lifestyle changes can you make to improve your score and reduce your risk?

Scores of 3 to 5 for each section: Your health-related behaviors are risky. What lifestyle changes can you make to improve your score in this area of health and reduce your risk?

Scores of 0 to 2 for each section: You may be taking serious and unnecessary risks with your health and, possibly, the health of others. What lifestyle changes can you make to improve your score and reduce your risk?

Source: Based on *Healthstyle: A self-test.* Hyattsville, MD: U.S. Public Health Service, 1981.

Eat wiser - lower fat and sugar intake.
Get back my brisk walking daily routine
Get yoga into my routine - schedule.
Hopefully this will help with stress
management.

I do believe in safety & the only smoking
I get is second hand smoke. It has been over
4 years since I have had a half a glass of
wine.
So food and exercise are my biggies!!

Chapter 1

SELF-ASSESSMENT 2 Personal Health History

Being aware of your family's health history, especially which relatives had or have serious chronic diseases or inherited conditions, can help you and your physician assess your risk of such diseases or conditions. As a result of having this information, you can make choices concerning your lifestyle now that may reduce the likelihood of developing these health problems in the future.

To compile your personal health history and design a health history diagram, start with your own health and that of your brothers and sisters. Then indicate health conditions that affect your mother and father and their brothers and sisters. After completing health information for that generation, collect information about your grandparents' health. You may be aware of some family members' health problems, such as heart disease, obesity, drug addiction, or mental health conditions. In other instances, however, you will need to speak with your relatives to determine whether they have or had diseases or conditions such as prostate or breast cancer, diabetes, hypertension, liver disease, and so on. If you are adopted or cannot find information about individual family members, you may have to leave blanks.

A sample family health history diagram is shown in this assessment. Note that it has spaces for a person to fill in his or her personal health and the health of siblings, parents, aunts, uncles, and grandparents. Of course, your diagram will reflect your family's makeup. After developing your personal health history diagram, answer the following questions.

1. If a particular disease or condition occurs repeatedly in your family, it may be the result of inherited and/or lifestyle factors that are common within your family. Such repeated occurrences may indicate that your risk of the disease or condition is greater than average. Which serious health problems occur more than once in your family health history?

   _____

   _____

   _____

2. Which diseases or conditions in your family history do you think are related to lifestyle practices, such as food choices, lack of regular physical activity, or smoking?

   _____

   _____

   _____

3. Are you aware of actions you can take that may reduce your risk of developing the health problems that often affect or have affected members of your family? If so, list those actions.

   _____

   _____

   _____

4. The course of many diseases and conditions is influenced by lifestyle factors. Your physician can help you determine such factors. Therefore, consider discussing your family health history with your physician. Your physician can also provide advice concerning steps you can take to reduce your risk of developing the health problems that affect or have affected members of your family.

Family Health History Example

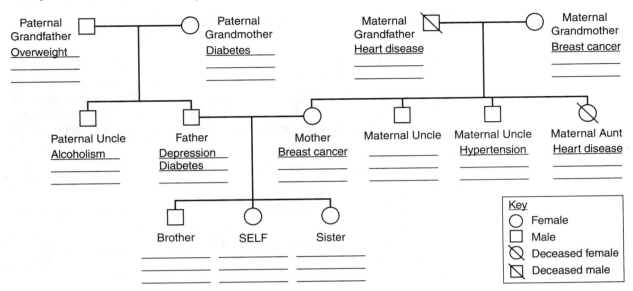

Chapter 1

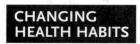 Model Activity for Better Health

This critical thinking feature describes a useful model of a decision-making process. The first part of the model involves deciding to change a health-related behavior; the second part describes implementing the behavioral change. To practice making responsible health-related decisions, complete the "Changing Health Habits" activities in this student workbook. Chapter 1 (below) is already completed as an example of how to use this model.

Deciding to Change

1. **Identify the problem, goal, or question.**

   Example: I'm overweight. I know that being overweight increases my risk for diabetes, certain cancers, and heart disease.

2. **List the reasons you should make this change and the reasons you should not.** Assign each reason a point value from 1 to 5, with 5 being the highest (it has the most value to you) and 1 being the lowest (it has the least value to you).

Choices

Reasons to lose weight (pros):		Reasons not to lose weight (cons):	
Points	*Reasons*	*Points*	*Reasons*
3	Losing weight will reduce my risk of diabetes, certain cancers, and heart disease.	2	I'll have to spend money on new clothes.
5	Losing weight will improve the way my clothes fit.	2	I'll have to spend money to join a health club or weight loss group.
4	Losing weight will help me feel better about myself.	4	I'll have trouble keeping the weight off.
5	Losing weight will reduce my flab.	5	I can continue eating fatty and sugary foods.
17	Total	13	Total

3. **Draw a conclusion.** Add the scores in each category. If the score of the positive reasons (pros) is greater than the score of the negative reasons (cons), you likely think that a change is in your best interest. Also, you are probably motivated to make the change and are likely to succeed. However, if your cons outweigh your pros, you likely think that changing is not in your best interest at this time. You may not be motivated to make the change now. Study your list of pros and cons carefully, however, before making your final decision. You may decide to change even if your reasons not to change outrank your reasons to change.

Implementing the Change

1. **Set a target date to begin the new behavior or reach the goal.** Depending on the type of decision, a behavior change could involve setting a beginning date and a goal date. For example, you could decide to lose 10 pounds by May 31st, then begin changing your eating and physical activity patterns tomorrow.

2. **Identify and list the factors that will help you reach your goal and those that will stand in the way of reaching your goal.**

   Factors that help
   My roommate has also decided to lose weight.
   I just got a check for my birthday to buy a new outfit when I lose 10 pounds.
   My student fees include the use of the health facility.

Factors that hinder

My mother insists that I eat a lot of food when I visit.

My roommate keeps lots of high-calorie snacks in the house.

I'm so busy that finding a time to exercise is difficult.

3. **Prepare an action plan for making the change.** An action plan specifies how you will change your behavior to meet your goal.

   a. **Identify alternative methods for reaching your goal.**

   Example

   > **Alternative 1:** Consume a 1,200-calorie diet that consists of eating only one meal a day and drinking a diet supplement for breakfast and lunch.
   >
   > **Alternative 2:** Consume a 1,200-calorie diet that permits three nutritious low-fat meals daily.
   >
   > **Alternative 3:** Consume a 1,200-calorie low-fat diet and increase exercise by 30 minutes a day.
   >
   > **Alternative 4:** Go to a weight loss clinic for help.

   b. **Gather information about each method.** Seek information that supports and criticizes each method. (People tend to gather data that only support what they think they want to do.) Ask yourself questions to guide your information gathering.

   Example: How long do people who reduce their caloric intake without exercising keep the weight off? By which method am I more likely to lose weight fastest? Is it better for my health to lose weight as quickly as possible, or does the length of time not matter? What changes will I have to make in my life if I decide to eat more nutritious foods and exercise? Are diet supplement drinks safe? Where can I find information about the caloric content of foods?

   c. **Choose the method that fits your situation best.**

   Example: After researching alternative methods, you decide to follow a 1,200-calorie-per-day, low-fat diet and increase the amount of exercise you engage in each day.

   d. **Consider the factors that can help or hinder your effort to change (see step 2).** What can you do that will take advantage of the helps and minimize the hindrances? For example, keep plenty of low-calorie snacks on hand to avoid being tempted by your roommate's supply of high-calorie munchies. Also, discuss the situation with your roommate to enlist his or her support in your effort.

4. **Change the lifestyle behavior that you have decided to improve by implementing the action plan you developed in step 3.**

5. **Chart your daily progress toward your goal.** Track your progress on a regular basis. Recording your weight once a week, for example, may be helpful. Are you losing weight?

6. **Evaluate how effective you were in reaching your goal.** Did your plan work? What can you learn from the experience?

   Example: You lost 5 pounds instead of 10 pounds. What seemed to keep you from reaching your goal? What can you do differently that might help you succeed? Do you need more time to lose weight, or do you need to reevaluate your decision?

Chapter 2

SELF-ASSESSMENT The Self-Esteem Inventory

If the following statement describes how you usually feel, put a check in the column "Like Me." If the statement does not describe how you usually feel, put a check in the column "Unlike Me."

There are no right or wrong answers. Read each statement quickly and answer the questions "off the top of your head."

Statement	Like Me	Unlike Me
1. I spend a lot of time daydreaming.	_____	_____
2. I'm pretty sure of myself.	_____	_____
3. I often wish I were someone else.	_____	_____
4. I'm easy to like.	_____	_____
5. My family and I have a lot of fun together.	_____	_____
6. I never worry about anything.	_____	_____
7. I find it very hard to talk in front of a group.	_____	_____
8. I wish I were younger.	_____	_____
9. There are lots of things about myself I'd change if I could.	_____	_____
10. I can make up my mind without too much trouble.	_____	_____
11. I'm a lot of fun to be with.	_____	_____
12. I get upset easily at home.	_____	_____
13. I always do the right thing.	_____	_____
14. I'm proud of my work.	_____	_____
15. Someone always has to tell me what to do.	_____	_____
16. It takes me a long time to get used to anything new.	_____	_____
17. I'm often sorry for the things I do.	_____	_____
18. I'm popular with people my own age.	_____	_____
19. My family usually considers my feelings.	_____	_____
20. I'm never unhappy.	_____	_____
21. I'm doing the best work that I can.	_____	_____
22. I give in very easily.	_____	_____
23. I can usually take care of myself.	_____	_____
24. I'm pretty happy.	_____	_____
25. I would rather associate with people younger than me.	_____	_____
26. My family expects too much of me.	_____	_____
27. I like everyone I know.	_____	_____
28. I like to be called on when I am in a group.	_____	_____
29. I understand myself.	_____	_____
30. It's pretty tough to be me.	_____	_____
31. Things are all mixed up in my life.	_____	_____
32. People usually follow my ideas.	_____	_____
33. No one pays much attention to me at home.	_____	_____
34. I never get scolded.	_____	_____
35. I'm not doing as well at work as I'd like to.	_____	_____
36. I can make up my mind and stick to it.	_____	_____
37. I really don't like being a man/woman.	_____	_____
38. I have a low opinion of myself.	_____	_____
39. I don't like to be with other people.	_____	_____
40. There are times when I'd like to leave home.	_____	_____

41. I'm never shy. _____ _____
42. I often feel upset. _____ _____
43. I often feel ashamed of myself. _____ _____
44. I'm not as nice-looking as most people. _____ _____
45. If I have something to say, I usually say it. _____ _____
46. People pick on me very often. _____ _____
47. My family understands me. _____ _____
48. I always tell the truth. _____ _____
49. My employer or supervisor makes me feel I'm not good enough. _____ _____
50. I don't care what happens to me. _____ _____
51. I'm a failure. _____ _____
52. I get upset easily when I am scolded. _____ _____
53. Most people are better liked than I am. _____ _____
54. I usually feel as if my family is pushing me. _____ _____
55. I always know what to say to people. _____ _____
56. I often get discouraged. _____ _____
57. Things usually don't bother me. _____ _____
58. I can't be depended on. _____ _____

Source: Ryden, Muriel B. (1978). An adult version of the Coopersmith Self-Esteem Inventory: Test-retest reliability and social desirability. *Psychological Reports, 43*:1189–1190. Used by permission.

Scoring the Self-Esteem Inventory

To determine your score, count the number of times your responses agree with the keyed responses below.

2. Like	22. Unlike	42. Unlike
3. Unlike	23. Like	43. Unlike
4. Like	24. Like	44. Unlike
5. Like	25. Unlike	45. Like
7. Unlike	26. Unlike	46. Unlike
8. Unlike	28. Like	47. Like
9. Unlike	29. Like	49. Unlike
10. Like	30. Unlike	50. Unlike
11. Like	31. Unlike	51. Unlike
12. Unlike	32. Like	52. Unlike
14. Like	33. Unlike	53. Unlike
15. Unlike	35. Unlike	54. Unlike
16. Unlike	36. Like	55. Like
17. Unlike	37. Unlike	56. Unlike
18. Like	38. Unlike	57. Like
19. Like	39. Unlike	58. Unlike
21. Like	40. Unlike	

The majority of the items measure self-esteem, but the eight items below that fall into the "Lie Scale" identify people who are trying to conceal their feelings about themselves. Count the number of times your responses to the questions listed agree with the responses shown below. If three or more responses agree, you may be trying to conceal feelings of low self-esteem.

1. Like	27. Like
6. Like	34. Like
13. Like	41. Like
20. Like	48. Like

How do you compare with other men and women taking this self-assessment? The average man obtains a score of 40; an average woman obtains a score of 39. Scores below 33 for men and 32 for women may indicate low self-esteem.

Chapter 2

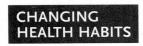

Are You Ready to Improve Your Psychological Health?

Do you need to change a behavior that relates to or affects your psychological health? For example, do you blame others for problems for which you should take responsibility? Do you eat too much fattening food or drink too much alcohol as a way of dealing with your problems? The "Deciding to Change" section of the worksheet can help you determine whether you are ready to alter your behavior to improve your psychological health. Use the "Implementing the Change" section of the worksheet if you decide to make the necessary changes.

Deciding to Change

1. Identify the problem, goal, or question.
2. List the reasons you should make this change and the reasons you should not.

Choices

Reasons to change thoughts
or behaviors (pros):

Points   *Reasons*

____   _____

____   _____

____   _____

____ Total

Reasons not to change thoughts
or behaviors (cons):

Points   *Reasons*

____   _____

____   _____

____   _____

____ Total

3. Draw a conclusion by adding the points in the pros section and then in the cons section. If the point total of the pros section is greater than the total of the cons section, you are probably ready to make a change that concerns your psychological health. If your cons outweigh your pros, you may not be motivated to make the change now. Study your list of pros and cons carefully, however, before making your final decision. You may decide to change even if your reasons not to change outrank your reasons to change.

Implementing the Change

1. Set a target date to begin the new behavior or reach the goal.
2. Identify and list the factors that will help you reach your goal and those that will stand in the way of reaching your goal.

   Factors that help: _____

   Factors that hinder: _____

3. Prepare an action plan for making the change.
   a. Identify alternative methods for reaching your goal.
   b. Gather information about each method.
   c. Choose the method that fits your situation best.
   d. Consider the factors that can help or hinder your effort to change (see step 2).
4. Change the lifestyle behavior that you have decided to improve by implementing the action plan that you developed in step 3.
5. Chart your daily progress toward your goal.
6. Evaluate how effective you were in reaching your goal.

Chapter 3

SELF-ASSESSMENT 1 How Much Stress Have You Had Lately?

To estimate the amount of stress that you have endured recently, indicate the number of occasions (to a maximum of four) that you have experienced the following in the past year.

Event	Number of Occasions	Points	Total
1. Death of a spouse	____	87	____
2. Marriage	____	77	____
3. Death of a close relative	____	77	____
4. Divorce	____	76	____
5. Marital separation	____	74	____
6. Pregnancy, or fathered a pregnancy	____	64	____
7. Death of a close friend	____	68	____
8. Personal injury or illness	____	65	____
9. Loss of your job	____	62	____
10. Breakup of a marital engagement or a steady relationship	____	60	____
11. Sexual difficulties	____	58	____
12. Marital reconciliation	____	58	____
13. Major change in self-concept	____	57	____
14. Major change in health or behavior of a family member	____	56	____
15. Engagement to be married	____	54	____
16. Major change in financial status	____	53	____
17. Major change in the use of drugs (other than alcohol)	____	52	____
18. Mortgage or loan of less than $10,000	____	52	____
19. Entered college	____	50	____
20. A new family member	____	50	____
21. A conflict or change in values	____	50	____
22. Change to a different line of work	____	50	____
23. A major change in the number of arguments with spouse	____	50	____
24. Change to a new school		50	____
25. A major change in amount of independence and responsibility	____	49	____
26. A major change in responsibilities at work	____	47	____
27. A major change in the use of alcohol	____	46	____
28. Revised personal habits	____	45	____
29. Being in trouble with school administration	____	44	____
30. A major change in social activities	____	43	____

Event	Number of Occasions	Points	Total
31. Holding a job while attending school	＿＿	43	＿＿
32. Change of residence or living conditions	＿＿	42	＿＿
33. A major change in working hours or conditions	＿＿	42	＿＿
34. Trouble with in-laws	＿＿	42	＿＿
35. Your spouse beginning or stopping work outside the home	＿＿	41	＿＿
36. Change in dating habits	＿＿	41	＿＿
37. A change involving your major field of study	＿＿	41	＿＿
38. An outstanding personal achievement	＿＿	40	＿＿
39. Trouble with your boss	＿＿	38	＿＿
40. A major change in amount of participation in school activities	＿＿	38	＿＿
41. A major change in type and/or amount of recreation	＿＿	37	＿＿
42. A major change in religious activities	＿＿	36	＿＿
43. A major change in sleeping habits	＿＿	34	＿＿
44. A trip or vacation	＿＿	33	＿＿
45. A major change in eating habits	＿＿	30	＿＿
46. A major change in number of family get-togethers	＿＿	26	＿＿
47. Found guilty of minor violations of the law	＿＿	22	＿＿

Multiply the number of occasions times the point value for each event. Add the scores.

TOTAL POINTS ＿＿＿＿＿＿

Your degree of stress is low if your score is lower than 347. If your score is higher than 1435, you are under a high degree of stress.

Source: "The influence of recent life experiences on the health of college students." Reprinted from *Journal of Psychosomatic Research*, 19:87–98 with permission from Elsevier.

Chapter 3

SELF-ASSESSMENT 2 ## K6 Serious Psychological Distress Assessment

Answer the following questions by checking the box that best applies.

During the past 30 days, how often did you feel?	All of the time 4	Most of the time 3	Some of the time 2	A little of the time 1	None of the time 0
So sad that nothing could cheer you up?					
Nervous?					
Restless or fidgety?					
Hopeless?					
That everything was an effort?					
Worthless?					
Total?					

Scoring: To score the K6, add the points for each of the questions together. Scores can range from 0 to 24. A threshold of 13 or more points indicates a high degree of distress and possibility of serious mental illness.

Source: National Center for Health Statistics (reviewed 2007). Serious psychological distress. Retrieved June 15, 2007, from http://www.cdc.gov/nchs/datawh/nchdefs/seriouspsydistress.htm.

Chapter 3

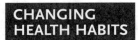 Taking Steps to Reduce Your Stress

Follow the steps of the decision-making and implementation model to identify and change a health-related habit that contributes to your level of stress. For example, do you work too many hours per week? Are you in a relationship that causes you continual stress? Are you trying to take care of your home and family with no help while going to school and working part-time?

Deciding to Change

1. Identify the problem, goal, or question.
2. List the reasons you should make this change and the reasons you should not.

Choices

Reasons to change behaviors (pros):		Reasons not to change behaviors (cons):	
Points	*Reasons*	*Points*	*Reasons*
____	_____	____	_____
____	_____	____	_____
____	_____	____	_____
____ Total		____ Total	

3. Draw a conclusion by adding the points in the pros section and then in the cons section. If the point total of the pros section is greater than the total of the cons section, you are probably ready to make a change in your life that reduces stress. If your cons outweigh your pros, you may not be motivated to make the change now. Study your list of pros and cons carefully, however, before making your final decision. You may decide to change even if your reasons not to change outrank your reasons to change.

Implementing the Change

1. Set a target date to begin the new behavior or reach the goal.
2. Identify and list the factors that will help you reach your goal and those that will stand in the way of reaching your goal.
   Factors that help: _____
   Factors that hinder: _____
3. Prepare an action plan for making the change.
   a. Identify alternative methods for reaching your goal.
   Alternative 1: _____
   Alternative 2: _____
   Alternative 3: _____
   Alternative 4: _____
   b. Gather information about each method.
   c. Choose the method that fits your particular situation best.
   d. Consider the factors that can help or hinder your effort to change (see step 2).
4. Change the lifestyle behavior that you have decided to improve by implementing the action plan you developed in step 3.
5. Chart your daily progress toward your goal.
6. Evaluate how effective you were in reaching your goal.

Chapter 4

SELF-ASSESSMENT 1 Assessing Your Anger

Anger can interfere with the ability to manage conflicts constructively. By becoming more aware of the situations that make you angry, your typical responses to these situations, and the consequences of your behavior, you may be able to identify and modify the destructive elements of your anger.

1. Keep a daily "anger journal" for at least a week.
   a. Record the time and date of the events that precipitated your anger.
   b. Describe the anger-evoking situations.
   c. For each of the events listed above, rate the intensity of your anger on a scale of 1 to 10, with 10 being the highest level of anger.
   d. Describe how you behaved before, during, and after each episode of anger.
   e. Describe how you feel after each angry episode and identify at least one consequence of your behavior.
2. Review your anger journal to see if there is a pattern of behavior, then complete the following statements.
   a. I frequently display anger when . . .
   b. When I am angry, I act . . .
   c. After most angry episodes, I feel . . .
3. Answer the following questions to assess the impact of your anger.
   a. Did my anger interfere with my ability to get along with others or perform my work?
   b. Did I use my anger to hurt others, physically or psychologically?
   c. Did my anger provoke others to hurt me, physically or psychologically?
4. If your angry responses threaten your health and well-being, consider taking a class to learn conflict management skills or obtain professional mental health counseling.

Source: Adapted from Napoli, V., Killbride, J. M., & Tebbs, D. E. (1996). *Adjustment and Growth in a Changing World, 5th edition.* Reprinted with permission of Wadsworth, a division of Thomson Learning; www.thomsonrights.com. Fax 800-730-2215.

Chapter 4

SELF-ASSESSMENT 2   Am I in an Abusive Intimate Relationship?

Read the following statements and indicate whether you agree or disagree with them. Draw a circle around your answer. Your responses can help you assess whether you are in an abusive intimate relationship.

1. My partner often embarrasses me in front of others.	Yes	No
2. My partner often criticizes my appearance, belittles my accomplishments, or makes fun of my ideas.	Yes	No
3. My partner frequently uses threats to make me to do what he/she wants.	Yes	No
4. My partner has told me that I'm worthless without him/her.	Yes	No
5. When my partner physically hurts me, he/she apologizes or says, "It was an accident," or "I didn't mean to hurt you."	Yes	No
6. My partner frequently has trouble controlling his/her anger.	Yes	No
7. My partner often makes me feel guilty when I want to spend time away from him/her.	Yes	No
8. My partner mistreats me when he/she gets drunk or high on drugs.	Yes	No
9. My partner usually blames me for his/her problems.	Yes	No
10. My partner pressures me for sex when I don't want it.	Yes	No
11. I often think about breaking up with my partner, but I don't because I'm afraid of what he/she might do to me or to himself/herself.	Yes	No
12. My friends and family members have told me that my partner is abusing me.	Yes	No
13. When I'm with others, I usually make excuses for my partner's abusive behavior.	Yes	No
14. I often sacrifice what I would like to do because I'm afraid of how my partner will respond if I don't follow his/her plans.	Yes	No
15. I often avoid saying or doing things that might anger my partner because I'm afraid that he/she will hurt me.	Yes	No

If you agreed with any of these statements, you may be in an abusive relationship. If you're not sure that your partner is abusive, seek counseling from a licensed professional therapist. If you are afraid of your partner, get help immediately. Contact your campus counseling center or a local domestic violence intervention center listed in your "Yellow Pages" phone book. The phone number for the National Domestic Violence Hotline is 1-800-799-7233.

Chapter 4

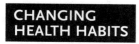 **Can You Reduce Your Risk of Violence?**

Follow the steps of the decision-making and implementation model to identify and change a health-related habit that contributes to your risk of violence. For example, do you ignore basic security measures? Are you involved in an abusive relationship that you feel hopeless about improving or terminating? Does your work, family, and college schedule force you to be exposed to risky situations and places?

Deciding to Change

1. Identify the problem, goal, or question.
2. List the reasons you should make this change and the reasons you should not.

Choices

Reasons to change behaviors (pros):		Reasons not to change behaviors (cons):	
Points	*Reasons*	*Points*	*Reasons*
____	_____	____	_____
____	_____	____	_____
____	_____	____	_____
____ Total		____ Total	

3. Draw a conclusion by adding the points in the pros section and then in the cons section. If the point total of the pros section is greater than the total of the cons section, you are probably ready to make a change in your life that reduces your risk of violence. If your cons outweigh your pros, you may not be motivated to make the change now. Study your list of pros and cons carefully, however, before making your final decision. You may decide to change even if your reasons not to change outrank your reasons to change.

Implementing the Change

1. Set a target date to begin the new behavior or reach the goal.
2. Identify and list the factors that will help you reach your goal and those that will stand in the way of reaching your goal.

   Factors that help: _____

   Factors that hinder: _____

3. Prepare an action plan for making the change.

   a. Identify alternative methods for reaching your goal.

   Alternative 1: _____

   Alternative 2: _____

   Alternative 3: _____

   Alternative 4: _____

   b. Gather information about each method.

   c. Choose the method that fits your particular situation best.

   d. Consider the factors that can help or hinder your effort to change (see step 2).

4. Change the lifestyle behavior that you have decided to improve by implementing the action plan you developed in step 3.

5. Chart your daily progress toward your goal.

6. Evaluate how effective you were in reaching your goal.

Chapter 5

SELF-ASSESSMENT 1 Contraceptive Comfort and Confidence Scale

The following series of questions, which are adapted from the Contraceptive Comfort and Confidence Scale, is designed to help you assess whether the method of contraception that you are using or may be considering for future use is or will be effective for you.

With regard to the method of birth control you are currently using or are considering using, answer YES or NO to the following questions:

1. Have you had problems using this method before?
2. Are you afraid of using this method?
3. Would you really rather not use this method?
4. Will you have trouble remembering to use this method?
5. Have you ever become pregnant using this method? (Or, has your partner ever become pregnant using this method?)
6. Will you have trouble using this method correctly?
7. Do you still have unanswered questions about this method?
8. Does this method make menstrual periods longer or more painful?
9. Does this method cost more than you can afford?
10. Could this method cause you or your partner to have serious complications?
11. Are you opposed to this method because of religious beliefs?
12. Is your partner opposed to this method?
13. Are you using this method without your partner's knowledge?
14. Will using this method embarrass your partner?
15. Will using this method embarrass you?
16. Will you enjoy intercourse less because of this method?
17. Will your partner enjoy intercourse less because of this method?
18. If this method interrupts lovemaking, will you avoid using it?
19. Has a nurse or doctor ever told you (or your partner) not to use this method?
20. Is there anything about your personality that could lead you to use this method incorrectly?
21. Does this method leave you at risk of being exposed to HIV or other sexually transmissible infections?

Total number of YES answers: _____

Interpreting Your Score

Most individuals will have a few "yes" answers. Yes answers predict potential problems. If you have more than a few yes responses, you may want to talk to your physician, counselor, partner, or a friend. Talking it over can help you decide whether to use this method or how to use it so it will be effective. In general, the more yes answers you have, the less likely you are to use this method consistently and correctly.

In choosing a method of contraception, keep in mind that if you want a highly effective method of contraception and a method that is highly effective in preventing transmission of STIs, you may have to use two methods. Hence, any method of contraception (except abstinence, of course) should be combined with condom use for maximum protection against STIs.

Source: Adapted from Hatcher, R. A., Stewart, F., Trussell, J., Kowal, D., Guest, F., Stewart, G. K., & Cates, W. (1990). *Contraceptive technology: 1990–1992* (15th ed., rev.) (p. 150). New York: Irvington.

Chapter 5

SELF-ASSESSMENT 2 Attitudes Toward Timing of Parenthood Scale (ATOP)

Directions

Circle the response that most closely represents your feelings. The options are strongly agree (SA), agree (A), undecided (U), disagree (D), and strongly disagree (SD).

	SD	D	U	A	SA
1. The best time to begin having children is usually within the first two years of marriage.	1	2	3	4	5
2. It is important for a young couple to enjoy their social life first and to have children later in the marriage.	1	2	3	4	5
3. A marriage relationship is strengthened if children are born in the early years of marriage.	1	2	3	4	5
4. Women are generally happier if they have children early in the marriage.	1	2	3	4	5
5. Men are generally tied closer to the marriage when there are children in the home.	1	2	3	4	5
6. Most young married women lack self-fulfillment until they have a child.	1	2	3	4	5
7. Young couples who do not have children are usually unable to do so.	1	2	3	4	5
8. Married couples who have mature love for each other will be eager to have a child as soon as possible.	1	2	3	4	5
9. Couples who do not have children cannot share in the major interests of their friends who are parents, and are therefore left out of most social circles.	1	2	3	4	5
10. Children enjoy their parents more when the parents are nearer their own age; therefore, parents should have children while they are still young.	1	2	3	4	5
11. In general, research indicates that the majority of couples approaching parenthood for the first time have had little or no previous child care experience beyond sporadic baby-sitting, a course in child psychology, or occasional care of younger siblings. Considering your background preparation for parenthood, would you judge that you are well prepared for the parenting experience?	1	2	3	4	5

Items 1 through 10 are from the Attitudes Toward Timing of Parenthood Scale (Maxwell & Montgomery, 1969). Item 11 was an additional item constructed to determine perceived degree of preparation for parenthood.

Scoring: Response options that favor early parenthood receive the highest score (5 points), and those that favor delayed parenthood receive the lowest score (1 point). The range of possible scores is from 10 to 50. Item number 2 is reverse scored, so if you choose option 4, change it to 2 (or vice versa); if you chose option 5, change it to 1 (or vice versa). Then sum the value of the options you selected for all items to compute your total score.

Reliability and validity: No reliability information was provided. The scale's developers, Maxwell and Montgomery (1969), reported that in an item analysis, each of the original 10-scale items discriminated significantly between upper- and lower-quartile groups. In their study of 96 married women, consistent attitudes and behavior were found; those who waited longer before having their first child scored lower on the ATOP.

Interpreting your score: Maxwell and Montgomery (1969) found that the following factors related to lower scores (favoring delay of parenting): higher age of respondent, higher education level and socioeconomic status, and having fewer children. Studies in the decade following publication of this measure reveal that women in the late 1970s and early 1980s were more likely than Maxwell and Montgomery's original sample to favor delayed parenthood (Knaub, Eversol, & Voss, 1981, 1983). In the 1983 study of 213 female students at a large midwestern university (Knaub, Eversoll, & Voss, 1983), the mean total score (on items 1 through 10) on the ATOP was 21.

Researchers using this measure typically present the percentage of respondents who agree and disagree with each item. Following is a table that summarizes the responses of 213 female students at a large midwestern university (Knaub, Eversoll, & Voss, 1983) and 76 male students from colleges in four states (Eversoll, Voss, & Knaub, 1983). Percentages for the response options "strongly agree" and "agree" are combined, as are the percentages for "disagree" and "strongly disagree."

ATOP Items by Percent of Respondents Agreeing and Disagreeing
(Refer to questions at the beginning of this assessment)

	Women			Men		
	Agree	Disagree	Undecided	Agree	Disagree	Undecided
Question 1	7.5	86.8	5.7	6.6	84.1	9.2
Question 2	78.8	10.8	11.3	76.0	11.8	13.2
Question 3	6.6	76.9	16.5	10.5	68.5	21.0
Question 4	5.2	72.7	22.1	5.3	58.0	36.5
Question 5	34.9	44.8	20.8	21.1	56.6	22.4
Question 6	8.9	81.7	9.4	7.9	72.4	19.7
Question 7	2.8	93.9	2.8	2.6	88.2	9.2
Question 8	4.3	84.4	11.3	9.2	81.6	9.2
Question 9	14.6	77.8	7.5	15.8	78.9	5.3
Question 10	15.6	71.2	13.2	19.8	64.5	15.8
Question 11	34.7	53.1	12.2			

Sources: Eversoll, D. B., Voss, J. H., & Knaub, P. K. (1983). Attitudes of college females toward parenthood timing. *Journal of Home Economics, 75*:25–29.

Knaub, P. K., Eversoll, D. B., & Voss, J. H. (1981). Student attitudes toward parenthood: Implications for curricula in the 1980s. *Journal of Home Economics, 73*:34–37.

Knaub, P. K., Eversoll, D. B., & Voss, J. H. (1983). Is parenthood a desirable adult role? An assessment of attitudes held by contemporary women. *Sex Roles, 9*:355–362. Reprinted with kind permission from Springer Science and Business Media and Patricia K. Knaub.

Maxwell, J. W., & Montgomery, J. E. (1969). Societal pressure toward early parenthood. *Family Coordinator, 18*:340–344.

Chapter 5

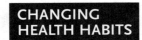 Do You Want to Improve Your Reproductive Health?

Do you need to change a behavior that relates to or affects your reproductive health? For example, if you are sexually active, are you using contraception irregularly, risking pregnancy? Are you using a method that does not provide the level of protection you desire? The "Deciding to Change" section of the Changing Health Habits worksheet can help you determine whether you are ready to alter your behaviors to improve your reproductive health. Use the "Implementing the Change" section of the worksheet if you decide to make the necessary changes.

Deciding to Change

1. Identify the problem, goal, or question.
2. List the reasons you should make this change and the reasons you should not.

Choices

Reasons to change behaviors (pros):   Reasons not to change behaviors (cons):
Points   *Reasons*   *Points*   *Reasons*

_____   _____   _____   _____
         _____   _____
_____   _____   _____   _____
         _____   _____
_____ Total   _____ Total

3. Draw a conclusion by adding the points in the pros section and then in the cons section. If the point total of the pros section is greater than the total of the cons section, you are probably ready to make a change in your life that improves your reproductive health. If your cons outweigh your pros, you may not be motivated to make the change now. Study your list of pros and cons carefully, however, before making your final decision. You may decide to change even if your reasons not to change outrank your reasons to change.

Implementing the Change

1. Set a target date to begin the new behavior or reach the goal.
2. Identify and list the factors that will help you reach your goal and those that will stand in the way of reaching your goal.

   Factors that help: _____

   _____

   Factors that hinder: _____

   _____

3. Prepare an action plan for making the change.

   a. Identify alternative methods for reaching your goal.

   Alternative 1: _____

   Alternative 2: _____

   Alternative 3: _____

   Alternative 4: _____

   b. Gather information about each method.

    c. Choose the method that fits your particular situation best.

    d. Consider the factors that can help or hinder your effort to change (see step 2).

4. Change the lifestyle behavior that you have decided to improve by implementing the action plan you developed in step 3.

5. Chart your daily progress toward your goal.

6. Evaluate how effective you were in reaching your goal.

Chapter 6

SELF-ASSESSMENT 1 ## Male Sexual Quotient Self-Assessment Questionnaire

This self-assessment addresses sexual function and satisfaction in men. It is designed to help men determine whether there are aspects of their sexual experience that could benefit from talking with their partner, consulting their physicians, and seeking treatment.

Answer this questionnaire honestly based on the last 6 months of your sex life, rating your answer as follows.

1 = Infrequently or rarely
2 = Sometimes
3 = Nearly 50% of the time
4 = Most of the time
5 = Always

1. Is your desire high enough to encourage you to initiate sexual intercouse?   _____
2. Do you feel confident in your ability of seduction?   _____
3. Do you feel that foreplay is enjoyable and satisfying for both you and your partner?   _____
4. Is your own sexual performance affected by your partner's sexual satisfaction?   _____
5. Can you maintain an erection sufficiently in order to complete sexual activity in a satisfactory way?   _____
6. After sexual stimulation, is your erection hard enough to ensure satisfying intercouse?   _____
7. Are you able to consistently obtain and maintain an erection whenever you have sexual activity?   _____
8. Are you able to control ejaculation so that sexual activity lasts as long as you want?   _____
9. Are you able to reach orgasm during sex?   _____
10. Does your sexual performance encourage you to enjoy sex more frequently?   _____

Male Sexual Quotient (MSQ) Scoring
. . . .

Total maximum score: 50

The MSQ equals total score multiplied by 2. Higher scores indicate greater sexual function and satisfaction with such function.

82–100   Highly satisfied: I am very sexually satisfied and enjoy my sex life to the maximum.
62–80   Partially satisfied: I enjoy sex, but there is some room for improvement.
42–60   Average: I am concerned that my sexual enjoyment really could be better.
22–40   Dissatisfied: I feel that my sex life does not give me enough satisfaction.
0–20   Highly dissatisfied: I am very concerned that I don't get any satisfaction from my sex life.

Source: Abdo, C. H. N. (2007). The Male Sexual Quotient: A brief, self-administered questionnaire to assess male sexual satisfaction. *Journal of Sexual Medicine,* 4:382–389. Reprinted with permission of Wiley-Blackwell.

Chapter 6

SELF-ASSESSMENT 2 Communication Patterns Questionnaire

This test not only evaluates your constructive communication patterns; it also gives you information about whether you and your partner engage in what is called the demand/withdraw pattern (also called the pursuer-distance pattern).

"Demand/withdraw" is a pattern in which one partner seeks closeness (i.e., she or he is demanding or pursuing) and the other partner responds, almost automatically, by withdrawing and seeking distance.

The demand/withdraw pattern can be very destructive for couples; what is so frustrating about demand/withdraw is that when one partner starts, by demanding or withdrawing, it is very difficult to resist reacting in a withdrawing or a demanding way. Some therapists call it a "mutual trap" because both partners are stuck in a pattern that is very hard to stop.

Directions

Rate each item on a scale of 1 to 9 (displayed below) in terms of how you and your partner typically deal with problems in your relationship.

	Very Unlikely								Very Likely

A. When some problem in the relationship arises,

1. both partners avoid discussing the problem. 1 2 3 4 5 6 7 8 9
2. both partners try to discuss the problem. 1 2 3 4 5 6 7 8 9
3. a. I try to start a discussion while my partner tries to avoid a discussion. 1 2 3 4 5 6 7 8 9
   b. my partner tries to start a discussion while I try to avoid a discussion. 1 2 3 4 5 6 7 8 9

B. During a discussion of a relationship problem,

1. both partners blame, accuse, and criticize each other. 1 2 3 4 5 6 7 8 9
2. both partners express their feelings to each other. 1 2 3 4 5 6 7 8 9
3. both partners threaten each other with negative consequences. 1 2 3 4 5 6 7 8 9
4. both partners suggest possible solutions and compromises. 1 2 3 4 5 6 7 8 9
5. a. I nag and make demands while my partner withdraws, becomes silent, or refuses to discuss the matter further. 1 2 3 4 5 6 7 8 9
   b. my partner nags and demands while I withdraw, become silent, or refuse to discuss the matter further. 1 2 3 4 5 6 7 8 9
6. a. I criticize while my partner defends herself. 1 2 3 4 5 6 7 8 9
   b. my partner criticizes while I defend myself. 1 2 3 4 5 6 7 8 9
7. a. I pressure my partner to take some action or stop some action, while my partner resists. 1 2 3 4 5 6 7 8 9
   b. my partner pressures me to take some action or stop some action, while I resist. 1 2 3 4 5 6 7 8 9

	Very Unlikely							Very Likely	

8. a. I express my feelings while my partner offers reasons and solutions.
1 2 3 4 5 6 7 8 9

   b. my partner expresses feelings while I offer reasons and solutions.
1 2 3 4 5 6 7 8 9

9. a. I threaten negative consequences and my partner gives in or backs down.
1 2 3 4 5 6 7 8 9

   b. my partner threatens negative consequences and I give in or back down.
1 2 3 4 5 6 7 8 9

10. a. I call my partner names, swear at him/her, or attack his/her character.
1 2 3 4 5 6 7 8 9

   b. my partner calls me names, swears at me, or attacks my character.
1 2 3 4 5 6 7 8 9

11. a. I push, shove, slap, hit, or kick my partner.
1 2 3 4 5 6 7 8 9

   b. my partner pushes, shoves, slaps, hits, or kicks me.
1 2 3 4 5 6 7 8 9

C. After a discussion of a relationship problem,

1. we each feel the other has understood our position.
1 2 3 4 5 6 7 8 9

2. we both withdraw from each other after the discussion.
1 2 3 4 5 6 7 8 9

3. we both feel that the problem has been solved.
1 2 3 4 5 6 7 8 9

4. neither of us is giving or generous to the other after the discussion.
1 2 3 4 5 6 7 8 9

5. we both try to be especially nice to each other.
1 2 3 4 5 6 7 8 9

6. a. I feel guilty for what I said or did while my partner feels hurt.
1 2 3 4 5 6 7 8 9

   b. my partner feels guilty for what s/he said or did while I feel hurt.
1 2 3 4 5 6 7 8 9

7. a. I try to be especially nice, act as if things are back to normal, while my partner acts distant.
1 2 3 4 5 6 7 8 9

   b. my partner tries to be especially nice, acts as if things are back to normal, while I act distant.
1 2 3 4 5 6 7 8 9

8. a. I pressure my partner to apologize or promise to do better, while my partner resists.
1 2 3 4 5 6 7 8 9

   b. my partner pressures me to apologize or promise to do better, while I resist.
1 2 3 4 5 6 7 8 9

9. a. I seek support from others (parent, friend, children).
1 2 3 4 5 6 7 8 9

   b. my partner seeks support from others (parent, friend, children).
1 2 3 4 5 6 7 8 9

Scoring and Evaluation

Mutual Constructive Communication Score

Calculate the scores as follows: (A2 + B2 + B4) minus (B1 + B3 + B10a + B10b). The range of answers is from −24 to +24. (You can have a negative number as a score.) The score is the sum of "positive communication styles" minus the sum of "negative communication styles." As you can imagine, people need to have more positive communication than negative communication to be happy. If your score is above zero, then you are doing well. If your score is zero or below, the research indicates that this may signal problems in communication that are leading your relationship into distressed territory. This doesn't prove that your relationship is on the rocks by any means, but it does tell you that your communication styles are a problem.

Demand/Withdraw Communication Scores

How much demand/withdraw communication is there in your relationship? To get this total, add A3a + A3b + B5a + B5b + B6a + B6b. The range is from 6 to 54. A score above 30 suggests this pattern is an issue in your relationship, according to an evaluation of the research.

Are You the Demander or the Withdrawer?

- To get your demander score, add A3a + B5a + B6a. The range for this score is from 3 to 27. If you scored above 18, then you may be the demander in the couple (which means that your partner may be a withdrawer).
- To get your withdrawer score, add A3b + B5b + B6b. The range for this score is from 3 to 27. Again, if you scored above 18, then you may be the withdrawer, and your partner may be a demander.

Although the demand/withdraw pattern can be difficult to overcome, it can be surmounted, in part, by recognizing it as a couple problem and not one person's fault.

One of the interesting things in the research on demand/withdraw patterns has to do with gender. The stereotype is that women are demanders, nagging for this or that, while men are the withdrawers, staying silent and ignoring her pleas. It turns out, however, that this is not always the case. Although women tend to be demanders more often, depending on the problem, the reverse pattern occurs (in which women are withdrawers and men demanders) about one-third of the time.

Mutual Avoidance and Withholding Score

This score can be calculated by adding A1 + C2 + C4. The range for this score is 3 to 27. High scores on this one, above 18, are cause for concern. In research by numerous psychological scientists, the avoidance and withholding stance in relationships is a sign of serious problems that require your attention. Mutual avoidance means that both partners withdraw whenever there is conflict. Even happy couples may be uncomfortable with conflict and use this strategy to avoid conflict. But over time this pattern can lead to distancing and leading "parallel lives" where there is no shared emotional life between the partners.

Other questions to which you responded are not included in the scoring above. They also reveal information about how partners interact. Blame, pressure, aggression, and guilt induction are other things you or your partner can do that will make matters worse, not better. You can detect these by looking at your responses to questions B1, B7a, B7b, and B8a and B8b, B10a and B10b, and 11a and 11b. Higher scores on these questions suggest that you and your partner try to manipulate each other in conflicts. Often these strategies are used to gain power.

On the other hand, "making nice" and even seeking outside support are constructive activities following conflict, as indicated in question C5, C9a, and C9b. Higher scores on these questions suggest that you are managing your conflicts well, which is important to sustaining a happy relationship.

Sources: Questionnaire by Andrew Christensen & Megan Sulloway, as reported in Christensen, A., & Heavy, C. L. (1993). Gender differences in marital conflict: The demand-withdraw interaction pattern. In S. Oskamp & M. Costanzo (Eds.), *Gender Issues in Contemporary Society.* Newbury Park: Sage. Reprinted with permission of Professor Andrew Christensen and Dr. Pepper Schwartz.

Directions: Rutter, V., & Schwartz, P. (1998). *The love test.* New York: The Berkeley Publishing Group (Perigee), pp. 100–101, 104–106.

Chapter 6

The Love Attitudes Scale

Listed below are several statements that reflect different attitudes about love. For each statement, fill in the response that indicates how much you agree or disagree with the statement. The items refer to a specific love relationship. Whenever possible, answer the questions with your current partner in mind. If you are not currently in a love relationship, answer the questions with your most recent partner in mind. If you have never been in love, answer in terms of what you think your responses would most likely be.

For Each Statement
....

1 = strongly agree with the statement
2 = moderately agree with the statement
3 = neutral—neither agree nor disagree
4 = moderately disagree with the statement
5 = strongly disagree with the statement

1. My partner and I have the right physical "chemistry" between us. _____
2. I feel that my partner and I were meant for each other. _____
3. My partner and I really understand each other. _____
4. My partner fits my ideal standards of physical beauty/handsomeness. _____
5. I believe that what my partner doesn't know about me won't hurt him/her. _____
6. I have sometimes had to keep my partner from finding out about other lovers. _____
7. My partner would get upset if he/she knew of some of the things I've done with other people. _____
8. I enjoy playing the "game of love" with my partner and a number of other partners. _____
9. Our love is the best kind because it grew out of a long friendship. _____
10. Our friendship merged gradually into love over time. _____
11. Our love is really a deep friendship, not a mysterious, mystical emotion. _____
12. Our love relationship is the most satisfying because it developed from a good friendship. _____
13. A main consideration in choosing my partner was how he/she would reflect on my family. _____
14. An important factor in choosing my partner was whether or not he/she would be a good parent. _____
15. One consideration in choosing my partner was how he/she would reflect on my career. _____
16. Before getting very involved with my partner, I tried to figure out how compatible his/her hereditary background would be with mine in case we ever had children. _____
17. When my partner doesn't pay attention to me, I feel sick all over. _____
18. Since I've been in love with my partner I've had trouble concentrating on anything else. _____
19. I cannot relax if I suspect that my partner is with someone else. _____

20. If my partner ignores me for a while, I sometimes do stupid things to try to get his/her attention back.   _____

21. I would rather suffer myself than let my partner suffer.   _____

22. I cannot be happy unless I place my partner's happiness before my own.   _____

23. I am usually willing to sacrifice my own wishes to let my partner achieve his/hers.   _____

24. I would endure all things for the sake of my partner.   _____

Scoring

Add your scores for the following groups of questions: 1–4, 5–8, 9–12, 13–16, 17–20, and 21–24. Each of these six groupings of questions corresponds to one of Lee's six styles of loving. Your lowest group score means that you most closely align yourself with that style of loving. Table 6-1 in *Essential Concepts for Healthy Living*, Fifth Edition, lists meanings and characteristics for each of Lee's six styles of loving.

1–4 = Eros
5–8 = Ludus
9–12 = Storge
13–16 = Pragma
17–20 = Mania
21–24 = Agape

Source: Hendrick, C., Hendrick, S. S., & Dicke, A. (1998). The love attitudes scale: Short form. *Journal of Social and Personal Relationships,* 15:147–159.

Chapter 6

CHANGING HEALTH HABITS Would a Behavior Change Improve Your Relationship?

Do you need to change a behavior that relates to or affects your relationships? For example, are your communication patterns ineffective with those close to you, such as your lover, spouse, or parents? Are you having trouble communicating effectively with other persons, such as a friend or your boss? Do you want to change those patterns so that you will be more effective in maintaining successful relationships? The "Deciding to Change" section of the Changing Health Habits worksheet can help you determine whether you are ready to alter your behaviors to improve your communication skills. Use the "Implementing the Change" section of the worksheet if you decide to make the necessary changes.

Deciding to Change

1. Identify the problem, goal, or question.
2. List the reasons you should make this change and the reasons you should not.

Choices

Reasons to change behaviors (pros):		Reasons not to change behaviors (cons):	
Points	*Reasons*	*Points*	*Reasons*
____	_____	____	_____
____	_____	____	_____
____	_____	____	_____
____	Total	____	Total

3. Draw a conclusion by adding the points in the pros section and then in the cons section. If the point total of the pros section is greater than the total of the cons section, you are probably ready to make a change in your life that improves your communications skills. If your cons outweigh your pros, you may not be motivated to make the change now. Study your list of pros and cons carefully, however, before making your final decision. You may decide to change even if your reasons not to change outrank your reasons to change.

Implementing the Change

1. Set a target date to begin the new behavior or reach the goal.
2. Identify and list the factors that will help you reach your goal and those that will stand in the way of reaching your goal.

    Factors that help: _____

    Factors that hinder: _____

3. Prepare an action plan for making the change.

    a. Identify alternative methods to reach your goal.

    Alternative 1: _____

    Alternative 2: _____

    Alternative 3: _____

    Alternative 4: _____

b. Gather information about each method.

c. Choose the method that fits your particular situation best.

d. Consider the factors that can help or hinder your effort to change (see step 2).

4. Change the lifestyle behavior that you have decided to improve by implementing the action plan you developed in step 3.

5. Chart your daily progress toward your goal.

6. Evaluate how effective you were in reaching your goal.

Chapter 7

SELF-ASSESSMENT Are You Dependent on Drugs?

Answer the following questions about your use and abuse of drugs.

	Yes	No
1. Have you used drugs other than those required for medical reasons?	———	———
2. Have you abused prescription drugs?	———	———
3. Do you abuse more than one drug at a time?	———	———
4. Can you get through the week without using drugs (other than those required for medical reasons)?*	———	———
5. Are you always able to stop using drugs when you want to?*	———	———
6. Do you abuse drugs on a continuous basis?	———	———
7. Do you try to limit your drug use to certain situations?*	———	———
8. Have you had "blackouts" or "flashbacks" as a result of drug use?	———	———
9. Do you ever feel bad about your drug abuse?	———	———
10. Does your spouse (or parents) ever complain about your involvement with drugs?	———	———
11. Do your friends or relatives know or suspect you abuse drugs?	———	———
12. Has drug abuse ever created problems between you and your spouse?	———	———
13. Has any family member ever sought help for problems related to your drug use?	———	———
14. Have you ever lost friends because of your use of drugs?	———	———
15. Have you ever neglected your family or missed work because of your use of drugs?	———	———
16. Have you ever been in trouble at work because of your use of drugs?	———	———
17. Have you ever lost a job because of drug abuse?	———	———
18. Have you gotten into fights while under the influence of drugs?	———	———
19. Have you ever been arrested because of unusual behavior while under the influence of drugs?	———	———
20. Have you ever been arrested while driving under the influence of drugs?	———	———
21. Have you engaged in illegal activities in order to obtain drugs?	———	———
22. Have you ever been arrested for possession of illegal drugs?	———	———
23. Have you ever experienced withdrawal symptoms as a result of heavy drug intake?	———	———
24. Have you had medical problems as a result of your drug use (e.g., memory loss, hepatitis, convulsions, bleeding, etc.)?	———	———
25. Have you ever gone to anyone for help for a drug problem?	———	———
26. Have you ever been in a hospital for medical problems related to your drug use?	———	———
27. Have you ever been involved in a treatment program specifically related to drug use?	———	———
28. Have you ever been treated as an outpatient for problems related to drug abuse?	———	———

Scoring This Assessment

If you answered "yes" to 6 or more of these questions (including "no" answers to questions 4, 5, and 7), you may have a drug abuse problem.

*Items 4, 5, and 7 are scored in the "no" or false direction.

Source: Skinner, H. A. The Drug Screening Test. *Addictive Behaviors*, 7:363–371. Copyright Elsevier 1982. Reprinted with permission.

Resources

If you are dependent on drugs, the following government agencies or private organizations may be able to provide you with help:

National Drug and Alcohol Treatment Referral Routing Service
1-800-662-HELP

Cocaine Anonymous World Services
3740 Overland Ave., Ste. C
Los Angeles, CA 90034
(310) 559-5833
E-mail: cawso@ca.org
http://www.ca.org

Nar-Anon Family Groups
22527 Crenshaw Blvd., #200B
Torrance, CA 90505
(310) 534-8188
1-800-477-6291
E-mail: naranonWSO@hotmail.com
http://nar-anon.org/index.html

Narcotics Anonymous World Services
P.O. Box 9999
Van Nuys, CA 91409
(818) 773-9999
E-mail: fsmail@na.org
http://www.na.org

National Council on Alcoholism and Drug Dependence
244 East 58th Street, 4th Floor
New York, NY 10022
Hope Line: 800-NCA-CALL (24-hour affiliate referral)
E-mail: national@ncadd.org
http://www.ncadd.org

National Institute on Drug Abuse
National Institutes of Health
6001 Executive Blvd., Rm. 5213
Bethesda, MD 20892-9561
(301) 443-1124
E-mail: Information@nida.nih.gov
http://www.nida.nih.gov

Chapter 7

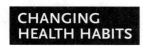
Are You Using Drugs Inappropriately?

Are you taking any drugs now, such as caffeine or much stronger drugs, that may be habit forming, may have negative health effects, and that were not prescribed by your health care practitioner? If you are using drugs inappropriately, follow the steps of the decision-making and implementation model to identify and change a drug-related habit.

Deciding to Change

1. Identify the problem, goal, or question.
2. List the reasons you should make this change and the reasons you should not.

Choices

Reasons to change behaviors (pros):		Reasons not to change behaviors (cons):	
Points	*Reasons*	*Points*	*Reasons*
_____	_____	_____	_____
_____	_____	_____	_____
_____	_____	_____	_____
_____ Total		_____ Total	

3. Draw a conclusion by adding the points in the pros section and then in the cons section. If the point total of the pros section is greater than the total of the cons section, you are probably ready to make a change in your life regarding a drug-related habit. If your cons outweigh your pros, you may not be motivated to make the change now. Study your list of pros and cons carefully, however, before making your final decision. You may decide to change even if your reasons not to change outrank your reasons to change.

Implementing the Change

1. Set a target date to begin the new behavior or reach the goal.
2. Identify and list the factors that will help you reach your goal and those that will stand in the way of reaching your goal.

    Factors that help: _____

    _____

    Factors that hinder: _____

    _____

3. Prepare an action plan for making the change.

    a. Identify alternative methods for reaching your goal.

    Alternative 1: _____

    Alternative 2: _____

    Alternative 3: _____

    Alternative 4: _____

    b. Gather information about each method.

    c. Choose the method that fits your particular situation best.

    d. Consider the factors that can help or hinder your effort to change (see step 2).

4. Change the lifestyle behavior that you have decided to improve by implementing the action plan you developed in step 3.

5. Chart your daily progress toward your goal.

6. Evaluate how effective you were in reaching your goal.

Chapter 8

SELF-ASSESSMENT 1   Why Do You Smoke?

Directions

Answer the following questions by circling O (often), S (sometimes), or N (never).

	Often	Sometimes	Never
Group 1			
I smoke to keep from slowing down.	O	S	N
I reach for a cigarette when I need a lift.	O	S	N
When I'm tired, smoking perks me up.	O	S	N
Group 2			
I feel more comfortable with a cigarette in my hand.	O	S	N
I enjoy getting a cigarette out of the pack and lighting up.	O	S	N
I like to watch the smoke when I exhale.	O	S	N
Group 3			
Smoking cigarettes is pleasant and enjoyable.	O	S	N
Smoking makes good times better.	O	S	N
I want a cigarette most when I am comfortable and relaxed.	O	S	N
Group 4			
I light up a cigarette when something makes me angry.	O	S	N
Smoking relaxes me in a stressful situation.	O	S	N
When I'm depressed I reach for a cigarette to feel better.	O	S	N
Group 5			
When I run out of cigarettes, it's almost unbearable until I get more.	O	S	N
I am very aware of not smoking when I don't have a cigarette in my hand.	O	S	N
When I haven't smoked for a while I get a gnawing hunger for a cigarette.	O	S	N
Group 6			
I smoke cigarettes automatically without even being aware of it.	O	S	N
I light up a cigarette without realizing I have one burning in an ashtray.	O	S	N
I find a cigarette in my mouth and don't remember putting it there.	O	S	N

Interpretation: Look at each group separately. If you answer "often" or "sometimes" to the questions in a particular group, that signifies one reason you smoke.

Reasons:

Group 1: Smoking gives you more energy.

Group 2: You like to touch and handle cigarettes.

Group 3: Smoking is a pleasure.

Group 4: Smoking helps you relax when you're tense or upset.

Group 5: You crave cigarettes; you are addicted to smoking.

Group 6: Smoking is a habit.

Refer to the Managing Your Health essay "Tips for Quitters" on page 216 of *Essential Concepts for Healthy Living* for strategies to quit that address each of these reasons you smoke.

Source: The National Cancer Institute. (1993). Learning why you smoke can teach you how to quit. Washington, DC: U.S. Department of Health and Human Services.

Chapter 8

SELF-ASSESSMENT 2 The CAGE Questionnaire

Circle your response.

Have you ever felt you ought to **C**ut down on your drinking?	Yes	No
Have people **A**nnoyed you by criticizing your drinking?	Yes	No
Have you ever felt bad or **G**uilty about your drinking?	Yes	No
Have you ever had an **E**ye-opener drink first thing in the morning, to steady your nerves or get rid of a hangover?	Yes	No

Scoring: One positive ("yes") response calls for further investigation. Two positive answers substantially increases the probability of alcohol dependence. Four positive responses suggests alcoholism.

Source: Ewing, J. (1984). Detecting alcoholism: The CAGE questionnaire. *JAMA,* 252(14): 1905–1907. Used by permission of the American Medical Association.

Resources
• •

If you are dependent on alcohol or tobacco, the following government agencies or private organizations may be able to provide you with help:

National Drug and Alcohol Treatment Referral Routing Service
1-800-662-HELP

Al-Anon Family Group Headquarters
1600 Corporate Landing Pkwy
Virginia Beach, VA 23454-5617
(888) 425-2666
E-mail: wso@al-anon.org
http://www.al-anon.alateen.org

Alcoholics Anonymous World Services
P.O. Box 459
New York, NY 10163
(212) 870-3400
http://www.aa.org

The American Lung Association
61 Broadway, 6th Floor
New York, NY 10006
(800) LUNGUSA
Lung HelpLine: 1-800-548-8252

National Institute on Alcohol Abuse and Alcoholism
5635 Fishers Ln., MSC 9304
Bethesda, MD 20892-9304
(301) 443-3860
E-mail: niaaaweb-r@exchange.nih.gov
http://www.niaaa.nih.gov

Centers for Disease Control and Prevention
National Center for Chronic Disease Prevention and Health Promotion
Office on Smoking and Health
1600 Clifton Rd.
Atlanta, GA 30333
1-800-232-4636
E-mail: tobaccoinfo@cdc.gov
http://www.cdc.gov/tobacco

National Council on Alcoholism and Drug Dependence
244 East 58th Street, 4th Floor
New York, NY 10022
Hope Line: 800-NCA-CALL (24-hour affiliate referral)
E-mail: national@ncadd.org
http://www.ncadd.org

Chapter 8

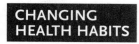
Do You Want to Change a Smoking or Drinking Habit?

Follow the steps of the decision-making and implementation model to identify and change a health-related habit that concerns your drinking of alcoholic beverages or your use of tobacco. For example, are you a heavy smoker who would like to smoke less or stop smoking cigarettes completely? Do you have drinking habits that you would like to change, such as drinking a six-pack in front of the TV every night, drinking on an empty stomach, or drinking too much at parties and sporting events?

Deciding to Change

1. Identify the problem, goal, or question.
2. List the reasons you should make this change and the reasons you should not.

Choices

Reasons to change behaviors (pros):
Points   *Reasons*

____   _____
____   _____
____   _____
____ Total

Reasons not to change behaviors (cons):
Points   *Reasons*

____   _____
____   _____
____   _____
____ Total

3. Draw a conclusion by adding the points in the pros section and then in the cons section. If the point total of the pros section is greater than the total of the cons section, you are probably ready to make a change in your life regarding a smoking or drinking habit. If your cons outweigh your pros, you may not be motivated to make the change now. Study your list of pros and cons carefully, however, before making your final decision. You may decide to change even if your reasons not to change outrank your reasons to change.

Implementing the Change

1. Set a target date to begin the new behavior or reach the goal.
2. Identify and list the factors that will help you reach your goal and those that will stand in the way of reaching your goal.

   Factors that help: _____
   _____
   Factors that hinder: _____
   _____

3. Prepare an action plan for making the change.

   a. Identify alternative methods for reaching your goal.

      Alternative 1: _____
      Alternative 2: _____
      Alternative 3: _____
      Alternative 4: _____

    b. Gather information about each method.

    c. Choose the method that fits your particular situation best.

    d. Consider the factors that can help or hinder your effort to change (see step 2).

4. Change the lifestyle behavior that you have decided to improve by implementing the action plan you developed in step 3.

5. Chart your daily progress toward your goal.

6. Evaluate how effective you were in reaching your goal.

Chapter 9

SELF-ASSESSMENT 1 Assessing the Nutritional Quality of Your Diet

Measure or estimate the amounts of everything you eat and drink for three days. For each day, record this information on a daily food record-keeping form (see the next page). To determine the nutritional value of your food items, you can look up the information in food composition tables that can be found in the back of nutrition textbooks or in the reference section of your college's library. The textbook's Web site (http://health.jbpub.com/healthyliving/5e) includes a content link in Chapter 9 for a Web site with a dietary analysis tool that you can use to determine the nutritional value of foods.

At the end of each day, add the amounts in each column and write the totals at the bottom of the form. Determine your average intake of calories and nutrients for that period. (Add the three daily totals for calories, then divide by 3. Do the same for each nutrient listed in the record-keeping form.) You can evaluate the nutritional quality of your diet by comparing your average intakes with the DRIs for those nutrients, which are shown in Appendix C.

1. Write a one-page description of the nutritional quality of your diet; in your summary, provide answers to the following questions:

   a. Did your average intake of calories and nutrients meet at least 70% of the DRIs for your age and gender?

   b. If your average intake of one or more nutrients did not meet 70% of the DRIs, which foods could you add to your diet to boost the amounts of the nutrient(s) you are lacking?

   c. For each of the three days, what percentage of your calories were from protein, fat, and alcohol?

   d. If the percentage of calories from fat exceeded 30%, which foods contributed to your high fat intake?

2. Do you need to make any changes to improve the nutritional quality of your diet? Would you like to eat more fruits or vegetables? Should you replace whole or reduced-fat (2%) milk with nonfat milk? Do you need more calcium or iron in your diet? Do you think you eat too much sugar, salt, or fat?

3. Use your responses to number 2 to complete the Changing Health Habits activity on page 52.

Daily Food Record

Name _____

Date _____

Food Item	Amount Eaten	Calories	Prot. (g)	Fat* (g)	Vit. A (RE)	Vit. C (mg)	Vit. E (mg)	Folate (μg)	Calcium (mg)	Iron (mg)
	Totals									

*No DRI

Total calories from alcohol _____

Chapter 9

SELF-ASSESSMENT 2 **Diabetes Risk Test***

Could you have diabetes and not know it? Over 18 million Americans have diabetes — and nearly one of three doesn't even know it! Take this test to see if you are at risk for having diabetes. Diabetes is more common in African Americans, Hispanic/Latinos, Native Americans, Asian Americans, and Pacific Islanders. If you are a member of one of these ethnic groups, you need to pay special attention to this test.

To find out if you are at risk, write in the points next to each statement that is true for you. If a statement is not true, write a zero. Then add all the points to get your total score.

	Yes	No
1. My weight is equal to or above that listed in the chart on the next page?	5 pts	0 pts
2. I am under 65 years of age and I get little or no exercise during a usual day?	5 pts	0 pts
3. I am between 45 and 64 years of age?	5 pts	0 pts
4. I am 65 years old or older?	9 pts	0 pts
5. I am a woman who has had a baby weighing more than nine pounds at birth?	1 pt	0 pts
6. I have a sister or brother with diabetes?	1 pt	0 pts
7. I have a parent with diabetes?	1 pt	0 pts

Total Points _____

Scoring 3–9 points

You are probably at low risk for having diabetes now. But don't just forget about it — especially if you are African American, Hispanic/Latino, Native American, Asian American, or Pacific Islander. You may be at higher risk in the future.

Scoring 10 or more points

You are at greater risk for having diabetes. Only your health care provider can determine whether you have diabetes. See your health care provider soon and find out for sure.

*This test is meant to educate and make you aware of the serious risks of diabetes. Only a medical doctor can determine whether you have diabetes.

Source: "Diabetes Risk Test" by American Diabetes Association. Copyright © 2008 American Diabetes Association. Reprinted with permission from The American Diabetes Association, www.diabetes.org.

At-Risk Weight Chart
Body Mass Index

Height in feet and inches without shoes	Weight in pounds without clothing
4'10"	129
4'11"	133
5'0"	138
5'1"	143
5'2"	147
5'3"	152
5'4"	157
5'5"	162
5'6"	167
5'7"	172
5'8"	177
5'9"	182
5'10"	188
5'11"	193
6'0"	199
6'1"	204
6'2"	210
6'3"	216
6'4"	221

If you weigh the same or more than the amount listed for your height, you may be at risk for diabetes.

Chapter 9

SELF-ASSESSMENT 3   Using the MyPyramid Plan

To complete this self-assessment, you will need to access the MyPyramid Plan via the Internet. When you open your Web browser, type http://www.mypyramid.gov/MyPyramid/index.aspx in the address window. This will take you to the U.S. Department of Agriculture's MyPyramid plan page. Insert your age in the appropriate box. In the other boxes, select your sex, weight, height, and the activity level that approximates your physical activity habits, most days of the week. Fill in the same information below.

Age _____ Sex _____ Weight _____ Height _____

Physical Activity Level _____

Click on the Submit button. The next page provides a personalized MyPyramid Plan that includes information about the number of calories you need to support your activity level as well as amounts of foods from each food group that you should eat daily. By following this food pattern, you are likely to obtain the nutrients you need each day and maintain your body weight.

Part I
....

Complete the following table with the information provided at your personal MyPyramid Plan page. Note that vegetables are divided into subgroups, and amounts for weekly consumption are recommended for each subgroup. Daily amounts are suggested for the other food groups.

Food Group	Amount of Food
Grains *	_____ ounces (refined grains)
	_____ ounces (whole grains)
Vegetables (daily)	_____ cups
Dark green (weekly)	_____ cups
Orange (weekly)	_____ cups
Dried beans and peas (weekly)	_____ cups
Starchy (weekly)	_____ cups
Other (weekly)	_____ cups
Fruits	_____ cups
Milk	_____ cups
Meat & Beans	_____ ounces
Oils (daily)	_____ teaspoons
Discretionary calories	Limit to no more than _____ calories daily

* At least half of your choices from the grains' group should be whole grains.

Part II

Use the MyPyramid Daily Food Record form to record everything you eat and drink for a day. You'll need to estimate the amounts of foods and beverages eaten and place that figure in the middle column. If you need to record information for more than one day, make copies of the form before you use it.

Name_____

MYPYRAMID DAILY FOOD RECORD		
Food/Beverage Item Consumed	**Amount Consumed** (Ounces/Cups)	**MyPyramid Plan Food Group**

Part III Self-Evaluation

1. According to your records, did you eat the recommended amounts of foods from each food group? ____ yes ____ no

   a. If you did not eat the recommended amounts, identify the food groups that had inadequate intakes.

2. Explain why this day's food intake was typical or unusual for you.

3. As a result of completing this activity, describe at least one step you can take to improve your daily food choices.

Chapter 9

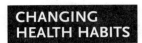 Are You Ready to Improve Your Diet?

After completing the summary for the nutritional assessment activity on pages 45 and 46, do you think you need to improve the nutritional quality of your diet? The "Deciding to Change" section of the Changing Health Habits worksheet can help you determine whether you are ready to improve your diet and what the health benefits might be if you do so. If you decide to change some food-related habits, use the "Implementing the Change" section of the worksheet to help you make your dietary changes.

Deciding to Change

1. Identify the problem, goal, or question.
2. List the reasons you should make this change and the reasons you should not.

Choices

Reasons to change behaviors (pros):		Reasons not to change behaviors (cons):	
Points	*Reasons*	*Points*	*Reasons*
____	_____	____	_____
____	_____	____	_____
____	_____	____	_____
____ Total		____ Total	

3. Draw a conclusion by adding the points in the pros section and then in the cons section. If the point total of the pros section is greater than the total of the cons section, you are probably ready to make a change in your life that improves the nutritional qulaity of your diet. If your cons outweigh your pros, you may not be motivated to make the change now. Study your list of pros and cons carefully, however, before making your final decision. You may decide to change even if your reasons not to change outrank your reasons to change.

Implementing the Change

1. Set a target date to begin the new behavior or reach the goal.
2. Identify and list the factors that will help you reach your goal and those that will stand in the way of reaching your goal.
    Factors that help: _____

    Factors that hinder: _____

3. Prepare an action plan for making the change.
    a. Identify alternative methods for reaching your goal.
        Alternative 1: _____
        Alternative 2: _____
        Alternative 3: _____
        Alternative 4: _____

b. Gather information about each method.

c. Choose the method that fits your particular situation best.

d. Consider the factors that can help or hinder your effort to change (see step 2).

4. Change the lifestyle behavior that you have decided to improve by implementing the action plan you developed in step 3.

5. Chart your daily progress toward your goal.

6. Evaluate how effective you were in reaching your goal.

Chapter 10

SELF-ASSESSMENT How Much Energy Do You Use Daily?

Use the following activity to estimate your daily caloric needs.

A. Estimating energy needs for basal metabolism:

1. Convert your body weight to kilograms. Since each pound equals about 2.2 kilograms, divide your weight in pounds by 2.2 to obtain your weight in kilograms.

    _____ weight in pounds ÷ 2.2 = _____ kilograms (kg)

2. To sustain its basal metabolic needs, the body needs about 1.0 calorie per kg of body weight per hour (men) or 0.9 calorie per kg of body weight per hour (women). To estimate the amount of calories you need for basal metabolism in an hour, multiply your body weight (kg) by 1.0 if you are male or 0.9 if you are female.

    _____ body weight (kg) × 1.0 or 0.9 = _____ calories per hour

3. To estimate the amount of calories you need for basal metabolism in a day, multiply the amount of calories you obtained in step 2 by 24 (hours in a day).

    _____ calories per hour × 24 hours = _____ calories per day (basal metabolism)

B. Estimating energy needs for physical activity:

4. To determine your energy needs for physical activity, you can keep records of every activity you perform during the day, and the time spent engaging in each activity. An easier, but less precise way to estimate your energy expenditures for physical activity is to use the following rule of thumb. To use this method, choose the category of physical activity in Table 10-A on the next page that best describes your usual physical activity level. For example, if you spend most of your day sitting while taking classes, studying, and watching TV, you probably have a sedentary level of activity. If you sit some of the time, but move around while working, you might rate your level of physical activity as light. If you are on your feet most of the time and engage in strenuous work such as lifting heavy objects, you are probably expending energy at the heavy level of intensity.

    My activity level is _____

5. Note the Activity Factor in Table 10-A for your level of intensity and gender. For example, if you are male, and you consider your overall physical activity pattern to be in the moderate range, your Activity Factor is 1.7.

    The Activity Factor for my gender and level of physical activity intensity is _____

6. Multiply your basal metabolic energy needs (the number of calories per day estimated in step 3) by the Activity Factor (step 5).

    ___ calories for basal metabolism × __ Activity Factor = ____calories for physical activity

7. To estimate the number of calories you expend each day for the thermic effect of food (TEF), multiply the number of calories determined in step 6 by 0.10.

_____ calories × 0.10 = ___ calories for TEF

8. To estimate your total energy needs for a day, add the number of calories determined in steps 6 and 7.

_____ calories for basal metabolism and physical activity
+ _____ calories for TEF

= _____ total calories

This is an estimation of the total number of calories you use each day. If you take in more calories than needed, they may be converted to body fat.

9. If you completed the assessment in Chapter 9, you were able to determine an average number of calories that you consumed during the three-day record-keeping period. Is your average caloric intake about the same, greater than, or less than the total number of calories that you need for a day?

____ about the same   ____ greater than   ____ less than

10. If you continue to consume this average amount of calories, explain what may happen to your body weight.

Table 10-A Determining Your Physical Activity Intensity Factor		Activity Factor	
Intensity	Physical Activity	Men	Women
Very light	Standing, sitting, driving, typing, sewing, cooking, playing cards or a musical instrument	1.3	1.3
Light	Walking on a level surface at 2.5 to 3.0 mph, carpentry, child care, golf, sailing, table tennis	1.6	1.5
Moderate	Walking 3.5 to 4.0 mph, gardening, carrying a load, cycling, skiing, tennis, dancing	1.7	1.6
Heavy	Walking uphill carrying a load; digging by hand; playing basketball, football, or soccer; climbing	2.1	1.9
Exceptionally heavy	Athletic training or participation in professional or world-class events	2.4	2.2

Source: Reprinted with permission from _Recommended dietary allowances_ (10th Ed.). Copyright © 1989 by the National Academy of Sciences. Courtesy of the National Academies Press, Washington, D.C.

Chapter 10

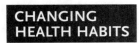 Altering Caloric Intake and Physical Activity

Do you need to lose or gain weight? The "Deciding to Change" section of the Changing Health Habits worksheet can help you determine whether you are ready to alter your caloric intake and physical activity level to gain or lose weight. If you decide to change some of your eating and physical activity habits, use the "Implementing the Change" section of the worksheet to help you make the necessary lifestyle changes.

Deciding to Change

1. Identify the problem, goal, or question.
2. List the reasons you should make this change and the reasons you should not.

Choices

Reasons to change behaviors (pros):
Points   *Reasons*

——   —————————————
——   —————————————
——   —————————————
——— Total

Reasons not to change behaviors (cons):
Points   *Reasons*

——   —————————————
——   —————————————
——   —————————————
——— Total

3. Draw a conclusion by adding the points in the pros section and then in the cons section. If the point total of the pros section is greater than the total of the cons section, you are probably ready to make the lifestyle changes necessary to lose or gain weight. If your cons outweigh your pros, you may not be motivated to make the change now. Study your list of pros and cons carefully, however, before making your final decision. You may decide to change even if your reasons not to change outrank your reasons to change.

Implementing the Change

1. Set a target date to begin the new behavior or reach the goal.
2. Identify and list the factors that will help you reach your goal and those that will stand in the way of reaching your goal.

   Factors that help: _____
   _____

   Factors that hinder: _____
   _____

3. Prepare an action plan for making the change.
   a. Identify alternative methods for reaching your goal.

   Alternative 1: _____
   Alternative 2: _____
   Alternative 3: _____
   Alternative 4: _____

   b. Gather information about each method.

   c. Choose the method that fits your particular situation best.

   d. Consider the factors that can help or hinder your effort to change (see step 2).

4. Change the lifestyle behavior that you have decided to improve by implementing the action plan you developed in step 3.

5. Chart your daily progress toward your goal.

6. Evaluate how effective you were in reaching your goal.

Chapter 11

SELF-ASSESSMENT 1 Cardiorespiratory Fitness: The Rockport
Fitness Walking Test™

This activity assesses cardiorespiratory (aerobic) fitness. To perform the test, you need a watch with a second hand to record your time, and you need to wear good walking shoes and loose clothes. You should have your physician's consent before undertaking this exercise test.

Instructions

1. Find a measured track or measure 1 mile using your car's odometer on a level uninterrupted road.
2. Warm up by walking slowly for 5 minutes.
3. Walk 1 mile as fast as you can, maintaining a steady pace. Note the time that you began walking.
4. When you complete the mile walk, record your time to the nearest second and keep walking at a slower pace. Count your pulse for 15 seconds and multiply by 4, then record this number. This gives you your heart rate per minute after your test walk.

   Heart rate at the end of a mile walk: _____ beats per minute

   Time to walk the mile: _____ minutes

5. Remember to stretch once you have cooled down.
6. To find your cardiorespiratory fitness level, refer to the appropriate Rockport Fitness Walking Test™ charts according to your age and sex. These show established fitness norms from the American Heart Association.

   Using your fitness level chart, find your time in minutes and your heart rate per minute. Follow these lines until they meet, and mark this point on your chart. This tells you how fit you are compared to other individuals of your sex and age category. Level 5 represents the highest fitness level.

   These charts are based on weights of 170 lb for men and 125 lb for women. If you weigh substantially less, your cardiovascular fitness will be slightly underestimated. Conversely, if you weigh substantially more, your cardiovascular fitness will be slightly overestimated.

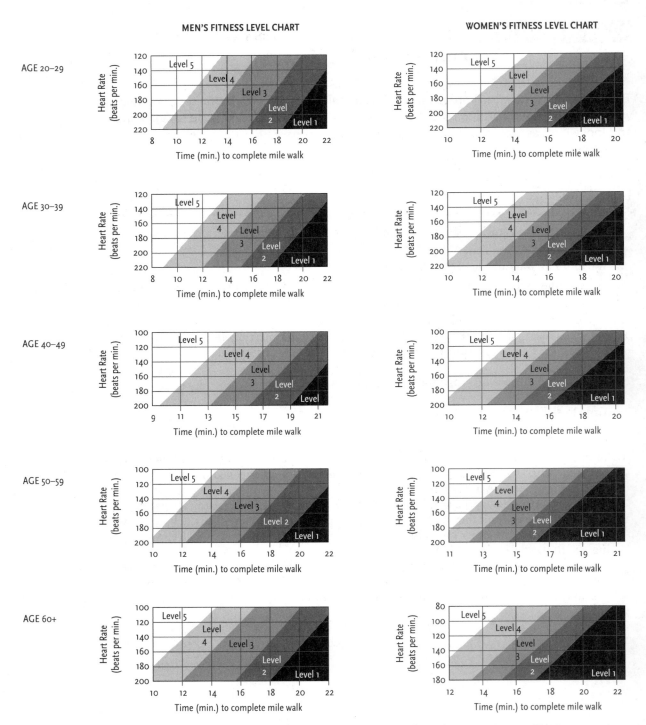

Chapter 11

SELF-ASSESSMENT 2   Partial Curl-Up Test

The partial curl-up test can help assess your muscular endurance. To prepare for the test, obtain a partner, a watch with a second hand, a comfortable mat to lie on, and a *metronome*, a device that produces a sound ("beat") evenly and regularly. To take the test, follow these instructions:

1. Lie on your back with your head resting on a mat, arms straight and parallel to the trunk, palms of the hands in contact with the mat. Have a partner mark a zero line at the tip of your middle finger when in the starting position.

2. Have your partner mark another line 10 cm (4 in) past the first line in the direction of your feet. Your arms should be fully extended when your fingertips are at the zero mark.

3. Your knees should be bent at a 90-degree angle with your legs hip-width apart. Keep your heels in contact with the mat. Perform the test with your shoes on.

4. Set a metronome to 50 beats per minute.

5. Slowly curl up your upper spine far enough so that the middle fingertips of both hands reach the 10-cm (4-in) mark. During the curl-up, the palms must remain in contact with the mat. Do not anchor your feet.

6. On the return phase, the shoulder blades and head must contact the mat, and the fingertips of both hands should touch the zero mark.

7. Perform the movement in a slow, controlled manner so that the time to perform the lifting and lowering stages of the curl-up is the same at a rate of 25 curl-ups per minute. Breathe normally throughout, exhaling during the upward motion.

8. Perform as many consecutive curl-ups as possible without pausing, to a maximum of 25 in the 1-minute period.

9. The test is terminated before 1 minute if you are:
   a. Experiencing undue discomfort.
   b. Unable to maintain the required cadence.
   c. Unable to maintain the proper curl-up technique (e.g., heels come off the floor) over two consecutive repetitions.

10. Record the number of partial curl-ups performed in the 1-minute period.

11. Use the following table to evaluate your score.

Age	Gender	Needs Improvement	Fair	Good	Very Good	Excellent
15–19	Male	≤15	16–20	21–22	23–24	25
	Female	≤11	12–16	17–21	22–24	25
20–29	Male	≤10	11–15	16–20	21–24	25
	Female	≤4	5–13	14–17	18–24	25
30–39	Male	≤10	11–14	15–17	18–24	25
	Female	≤5	6–9	10–18	19–24	25
40–49	Male	≤5	6–12	13–17	18–24	25
	Female	≤3	4–10	11–18	19–24	25
50–59	Male	≤7	8–10	11–16	17–24	25
	Female	≤5	6–9	10–18	19–24	25
60–69	Male	≤5	6–10	11–15	16–24	25
	Female	≤2	3–7	8–16	17–24	25

Source: From *The Canadian Physical Activity, Fitness, & Lifestyle Approach: CSEP-Health & Fitness Program's Health-Related Appraisal & Counseling Strategy 3E,* © 2003. Reprinted with permission from the Canadian Society for Exercise Physiology.

Chapter 11

SELF-ASSESSMENT 3 Push-Up Test for Muscular Endurance

The push-up test can help assess your muscular endurance. To take the test, follow these instructions.

Procedure

Men

- Assume the standard position for a push-up, with the body rigid and straight, toes tucked under, and hands about shoulder-width apart and straight under the shoulders.
- Lower the body until the elbows reach 90 degrees. Some prefer to place an object such as a paper cup beneath to touch.
- Return to the starting position with the arms fully extended.
- The most common error is not keeping the back straight and rigid throughout the entire push-up.
- Count the number of push-ups you can perform in one minute.
- See the accompanying table for your fitness level.

Women

Women tend to have less upper body strength and therefore should use the modified push-up position to assess their upper body endurance. The test is performed as follows:

- Directions are the same for women as for men, except that women should perform the test from the bent-knee position. Make sure that your hands are slightly ahead of your shoulders in the up position so that when you are in the down position, your hands are directly under the shoulders.
- Keep the back straight and rigid throughout the entire push-up.
- Count the number of push-ups you can perform in one minute.
- See the accompanying table to rate your muscular endurance.

Note: Women who wish to do full-body push-ups can rate their performances by using the table on page 66.

Muscular Endurance Ratings
1 Minute Push-Up

Males
Age

%	20–29	30–39	40–49	50–59	
99	100	86	64	51	
95	62	52	40	39	Superior
90	57	46	36	30	
85	51	41	34	28	
80	47	39	30	25	Excellent
75	44	36	29	24	
70	41	34	26	21	
65	39	31	25	20	
60	37	30	24	19	Good
55	35	29	22	17	
50	33	27	21	15	
45	31	25	19	14	
40	29	24	18	13	Fair
35	27	21	16	11	
30	26	20	15	10	
25	24	19	13	9.5	
20	22	17	11	9	Poor
15	19	15	10	7	
10	18	13	9	6	
5	13	9	5	3	Very Poor
n	1,045	790	364	172	

Total n = 2,371

Note: Norms are based on worksite wellness program participants.

Muscular Endurance Ratings
1 Minute Modified Push-Up

Females
Age

%	20–29	30–39	40–49	50–59	
99	70	56	60	31	
95	45	39	33	28	Superior
90	42	36	28	25	
85	39	33	26	23	
80	36	31	24	21	Excellent
75	34	29	21	20	
70	32	28	20	19	
65	31	26	19	18	
60	30	24	18	17	Good
55	29	23	17	15	
50	26	21	15	13	
45	25	20	14	13	
40	23	19	13	12	Fair
35	22	17	11	10	
30	20	15	10	9	
25	19	14	9	8	
20	17	11	6	6	Poor
15	15	9	4	4	
10	12	8	2	1	
5	9	4	1	0	Very Poor
n	579	411	246	105	

Total n = 1,341

Note: Norms are based on worksite wellness program participants.

Muscular Endurance Ratings
1 Minute Full Body Push-Up*

Females
Age

%	20–29	30–39	40–49	
99	53.0	48.0	23.0	
95	42.0	39.5	20.0	Superior
90	37.0	33.0	18.0	
85	33.0	26.0	17.0	
80	28.0	23.0	15.0	Excellent
75	27.0	19.0	15.0	
70	24.0	18.0	14.0	
65	23.0	16.0	13.0	
60	21.0	15.0	13.0	Good
55	19.0	14.0	11.0	
50	18.0	14.0	11.0	
45	17.0	13.0	10.0	
40	15.0	11.0	9.0	Fair
35	14.0	10.0	8.0	
30	13.0	9.0	7.0	
25	11.0	9.0	7.0	
20	10.0	8.0	6.0	Poor
15	9.0	6.5	5.0	
10	8.0	6.0	4.0	
5	6.0	4.0	1.0	
1	3.0	1.0	0.0	Very Poor

* Full body push-ups are generally used by law enforcement and public safety organizations. These norms are based on >1000 female U.S. Army soldiers who were tested in the 1990s by the U.S. Army.

Reprinted with permission from The Cooper Institute, Dallas, Texas, from *Physical Fitness Assessments and Norms for Adults and Law Enforcement*. Available online at http://www.cooperinstitute.org.

Chapter 11

SELF-ASSESSMENT 4 Sit-and-Reach Test for Flexibility
Assessment

The sit-and-reach test can help assess your flexibility. Read the following precautions, and if they do not apply, take the test.

Precautions

If any of the following apply, seek medical advice before performing the test.

- You are presently suffering from acute back pain.
- You are currently receiving treatment for back pain.
- You have ever had a surgical operation on your back.
- A health care professional told you to never exercise your back.

Procedure

Warm up. Stop the test if pain occurs. Do not perform fast, jerky movements.

Step 1:

Sit on the floor with your legs straight and knees together. Your toes should point upward toward the ceiling and rest against the side of a box.

Step 2:

Place one hand over the other. The tips of your two middle fingers should be on top of each other.

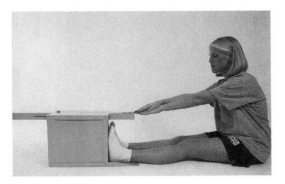

Step 3:

Slowly stretch forward without bouncing or jerking. Stop when tightness or discomfort occurs in the back or legs. Measure how far your hands reached on the top of the box.

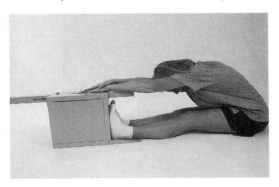

Step 4:

Repeat this test two more times and record scores.

First attempt   —————— points

Second attempt   —————— points

Third attempt   —————— points

How to score (average of 3 attempts)	
Reached well past toes and side of box	1 point; excellent
Reached just to toes	2 points; good
Up to 4 inches from toes (did not reach side of box)	3 points; fair
More than 4 inches from toes (did not reach side of box)	4 points; poor

Source: David Imrie. (1998). *Back power*. Toronto, Canada: Stoddart. Reprinted with permission of the author.

Total points = —————— divided by 3 = —————— points, which is rated as ——————.

Chapter 11

SELF-ASSESSMENT 5 Check Your Physical Activity and Heart Disease IQ

Test your knowledge about the effects that physical activity can have on your heart. Mark each statement true or false. Answers are on the following page.

1. Regular physical activity can reduce your chances of getting heart disease.   T   F

2. Most people get enough physical activity from their normal daily routines.   T   F

3. You don't have to train like a marathon runner to become more physically fit.   T   F

4. Exercise programs do not require a lot of time to be very effective.   T   F

5. People who need to lose some weight are the only ones who will benefit from regular physical activity.   T   F

6. All exercises give you the same benefits.   T   F

7. The older you are, the less active you need to be.   T   F

8. It doesn't take a lot of money or expensive equipment to become physically fit.   T   F

9. There are many risks and injuries that can occur with exercise.   T   F

10. You should consult a doctor before starting a physical activity program.   T   F

11. People who have had a heart attack should not start any physical activity program.   T   F

12. To help stay physically active, include a variety of activities.   T   F

How well did you do?

Answers to the Check Your Physical Activity and Heart Disease IQ Quiz

1. *True.* Heart disease is almost twice as likely to develop in inactive people. Being physically inactive is a risk factor for heart disease, along with cigarette smoking, high blood pressure, high blood cholesterol, and being overweight. The more risk factors you have, the greater your chance for heart disease. Regular physical activity (even mild to moderate exercise) can reduce this risk.

2. *False.* Most Americans are very busy but not very active. Every American adult should make a habit of getting at least 30 minutes of low to moderate levels of physical activity daily. This includes walking, gardening, and walking up stairs. If you are inactive now, begin by doing a few minutes of activity each day. If you only do some activity every once in a while, try to work something into your routine everyday.

3. *True.* Low- to moderate-intensity activities, such as pleasure walking, stair climbing, yard work, housework, dancing, and home exercises can have both short- and long-term benefits. If you are inactive, the key is to get started. One great way is to take a walk for 10 to 15 minutes during your lunch break, or take your dog for a walk every day. At least 30 minutes of physical activity every day can help improve your heart health.

4. *True.* It takes only a few minutes a day to become more physically active. If you don't have 30 minutes in your schedule for an exercise break, try to find two 15-minute periods or even three 10-minute periods. These exercise breaks will soon become a habit you can't live without.

5. *False.* People who are physically active experience many positive benefits. Regular physical activity gives you more energy, reduces stress, and helps you to sleep better. It helps to lower high blood pressure and improves blood cholesterol levels. Physical activity helps to tone your muscles, burns off calories to help you lose extra pounds or stay at your desirable weight, and helps control your appetite. It can also increase muscle strength, help your heart and lungs work more efficiently, and let you enjoy your life more fully.

6. *False.* Low-intensity activities — if performed daily — can have some long-term health benefits and can lower your risk of heart disease. Regular, brisk, and sustained exercise for at least 30 minutes, three to four times a week, such as brisk walking, jogging, or swimming, is necessary to improve the efficiency of your heart and lungs and burn off extra calories. These activities are called aerobic — meaning the body uses oxygen to produce the energy needed for the activity. Other activities, depending on the type, may give you other benefits such as increased flexibility or muscle strength.

7. *False.* Although we tend to become less active with age, physical activity is still important. In fact, regular physical activity in older persons increases their capacity to do everyday activities. In general, middle-aged and older people benefit from regular physical activity just as young people do. What is important, at any age, is tailoring the activity program to your own fitness level.

8. *True.* Many activities require little or no equipment. For example, brisk walking only requires a comfortable pair of walking shoes. Many communities offer free or inexpensive recreation facilities and physical activity classes. Check your shopping malls, as many of them are open early and late for people who do not wish to walk alone, in the dark, or in bad weather.

9. *False.* Under normal conditions, exercise does not involve many risks and injuries. However, the most common risk in exercising is injury to the muscles and joints. Such injuries are usually caused by exercising too hard for too long, particularly if a person has been inactive. To avoid injuries, try to build up your level of activity gradually, listen to your body for warning pains, be aware of possible signs of heart problems (such as pain or pressure in the left

or mid-chest area, left neck, shoulder, or arm during or just after exercising, or sudden light-headedness, cold sweat, pallor, or fainting), and be prepared for special weather conditions.

10. *True.* You should ask your doctor before you start (or greatly increase) your physical activity **if** you have a medical condition such as high blood pressure, have pains or pressure in the chest and shoulder, feel dizzy or faint, get breathless after mild exertion, are middle-aged or older and have not been physically active, or plan a vigorous activity program. If none of these apply, start slow and get moving.

11. *False.* Regular physical activity can help reduce your risk of having another heart attack. People who include regular physical activity in their lives after a heart attack improve their chances of survival and can improve how they feel and look. If you have had a heart attack, consult your doctor to be sure you are following a safe and effective exercise program that will help prevent heart pain and further damage from overexertion.

12. *True.* Pick several different activities that you like doing. You will be more likely to stay with it. Plan short-term and long-term goals. Keep a record of your progress, and check it regularly to see the progress you have made. Get your family and friends to join in. They can help keep you going.

Source: U.S. Department of Health and Human Services, National Institutes of Health, National Heart, Lung, and Blood Institute. Retrieved April 7, 2008, from http://www.nhlbi.nih.gov/health/public/heart/obesity/phy_act.htm.

Chapter 11

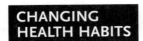 **Do You Want to Be More Physically Active?**

After completing the cardiorespiratory fitness assessment in the workbook, do you think you need to increase your physical activity level to become more fit? The "Deciding to Change" section of the Changing Health Habits worksheet can help you identify the health benefits of adding physical activity to your schedule and decide whether you are ready to do so. If you choose to increase your present level of physical activity, use the "Implementing the Change" section of the worksheet to help you.

Deciding to Change

1. Identify the problem, goal, or question.
2. List the reasons you should make this change and the reasons you should not.

Choices

Reasons to change behaviors (pros):

Points   *Reasons*

_____   _____

_____   _____

_____   _____

_____ Total

Reasons not to change behaviors (cons):

Points   *Reasons*

_____   _____

_____   _____

_____   _____

_____ Total

3. Draw a conclusion by adding the points in the pros section and then in the cons section. If the point total of the pros section is greater than the total of the cons section, you are probably ready to make a change that increases your level of physical activity. If your cons outweigh your pros, you may not be motivated to make the change now. Study your list of pros and cons carefully, however, before making your final decision. You may decide to change even if your reasons not to change outrank your reasons to change.

Implementing the Change

1. Set a target date to begin the new behavior or reach the goal.
2. Identify and list the factors that will help you reach your goal and those that will stand in the way of reaching your goal.

   Factors that help: _____

   _____

   Factors that hinder: _____

   _____

3. Prepare an action plan for making the change.

   a. Identify alternative methods for reaching your goal.

   Alternative 1: _____

   Alternative 2: _____

   Alternative 3: _____

   Alternative 4: _____

    b. Gather information about each method.

    c. Choose the method that fits your situation best.

    d. Consider the factors that can help or hinder your effort to change (see step 2).

4. Change the exercise-related behavior that you have decided to improve by implementing the action plan you developed in step 3.

5. Chart your daily progress toward your goal.

6. Evaluate how effective you were in reaching your goal.

Chapter 12

SELF-ASSESSMENT ## What is Your Risk of Developing Heart Disease or Having a Heart Attack?

In general, the higher your LDL level and the more risk factors you have (other than LDL), the greater your chances of developing heart disease or having a heart attack. Some people are at high risk for a heart attack because they already have heart disease. Other people are at high risk for developing heart disease because they have diabetes (which is a strong risk factor) or a combination of risk factors for heart disease. Follow these steps to find out your risk for developing heart disease.

Step 1: Check the following table to see how many of the listed risk factors you have; these are the risk factors that affect your LDL goal.

Major Risk Factors That Affect Your LDL Goal

- Cigarette smoking

- High blood pressure (140/90 mmHg or higher or on blood pressure medication)

- Low HDL cholesterol (less than 40 mg/dl)*

- Family history of early heart disease (heart disease in father or brother before age 55; heart disease in mother or sister before age 65)

- Age (men 45 years or older; women 55 years or older)

*If your HDL cholesterol is 60 mg/dl or higher, subtract 1 from your total count.

Even though obesity and physical inactivity are not counted in this list, they are conditions that need to be corrected.

Step 2: How many major risk factors do you have? If you have two or more risk factors in the bulleted list above, use the risk scoring tables at the end of this assessment (which include your cholesterol levels) to find your risk score. Risk score refers to the chance of having a heart attack in the next 10 years, given as a percentage. My risk score is _____%.

Step 3: Use your medical history, number of risk factors, and risk score to find your risk of developing heart disease or having a heart attack in the following table.

If You Have	You Are in Category
Heart disease, diabetes, or risk score more than 20%*	I. High Risk
2 or more risk factors and risk score 10–20%	II. Next Highest Risk
2 or more risk factors and risk score less than 10%	III. Moderate Risk
0 or 1 risk factor	IV. Low-to-Moderate Risk

*Means that more than 20 of 100 people in this category will have a heart attack within 10 years.

My risk category is _____.

Treating High Cholesterol
. . . .

The main goal of cholesterol-lowering treatment is to lower your LDL level enough to reduce your risk of developing heart disease or having a heart attack. The higher your risk, the lower your LDL goal will be. To find your LDL goal, see the bulleted list that follows for your risk category. There are two main ways to lower your cholesterol:

1. Therapeutic lifestyle changes (TLC): Includes a cholesterol-lowering diet (called the TLC diet), physical activity, and weight management. TLC is for anyone whose LDL is above goal.
2. Drug treatment: If cholesterol-lowering drugs are needed, they are used together with TLC treatment to help lower your LDL.

If you are in . . .

- **Category I, Highest Risk**, your LDL goal is less than 100 mg/dl. You will need to begin the TLC diet to reduce your high risk even if your LDL is below 100 mg/dl. If your LDL is 100 or above, you will need to start drug treatment at the same time as the TLC diet. If your LDL is below 100 mg/dl, you may also need to start drug treatment together with the TLC diet if your doctor finds your risk is very high—for example, if you had a recent heart attack or have both heart disease and diabetes.
- **Category II, Next Highest Risk**, your LDL goal is less than 130 mg/dl. If your LDL is 130 mg/dl or above, you will need to begin treatment with the TLC diet. If your LDL is 130 mg/dl or more after 3 months on the TLC diet, you may need drug treatment along with the TLC diet. If your LDL is less than 130 mg/dl, you will need to follow the heart-healthy diet for all Americans, which allows a little more saturated fat and cholesterol than the TLC diet.
- **Category III, Moderate Risk**, your LDL goal is less than 130 mg/dl. If your LDL is 130 mg/dl or above, you will need to begin the TLC diet. If your LDL is 160 mg/dl or more after you have tried the TLC diet for 3 months, you may need drug treatment along with the TLC diet. If your LDL is less than 130 mg/dl, you will need to follow the heart-healthy diet for all Americans.
- **Category IV, Low-to-Moderate Risk**, your LDL goal is less than 160 mg/dl. If your LDL is 160 mg/dl or above, you will need to begin the TLC diet. If your LDL is still 160 mg/dl or more after 3 months on the TLC diet, you may need drug treatment along with the TLC diet to lower your LDL, especially if your LDL is 190 mg/dl or more. If your LDL is less than 160 mg/dl, you will need to follow the heart-healthy diet for all Americans.

To reduce your risk for heart disease or keep it low, it is very important to control any other risk factors you may have, such as high blood pressure and smoking.

Lowering Cholesterol with Therapeutic Lifestyle Changes

TLC is a set of things you can do to help lower your LDL cholesterol. The main parts of TLC are:

- *The TLC diet.* This is a low-saturated-fat, low-cholesterol eating plan that calls for less than 7% of calories from saturated fat and less than 200 mg of dietary cholesterol per day. The TLC diet recommends only enough calories to maintain a desirable weight and avoid weight gain. If your LDL is not lowered enough by reducing your saturated fat and cholesterol intakes, the amount of soluble fiber in your diet can be increased. Certain food products that contain plant stanols or plant sterols (for example, cholesterol-lowering margarines) can also be added to the TLC diet to boost its LDL-lowering power.
- *Weight management.* Losing weight if you are overweight can help lower LDL and is especially important for those with a cluster of risk factors that includes high triglyceride and/or low HDL levels and being overweight with a large waist measurement (more than 40 inches for men and more than 35 inches for women).

- *Physical activity.* Regular physical activity (30 minutes on most, if not all, days) is recommended for everyone. It can help raise HDL and lower LDL and is especially important for those with high triglyceride and/or low HDL levels who are overweight with a large waist measurement.

Foods low in saturated fat include fat-free or 1% dairy products, lean meats, fish, skinless poultry, whole-grain foods, and fruits and vegetables. Look for soft margarines (liquid or tub varieties) that are low in saturated fat and contain little or no trans fat (another type of dietary fat that can raise your cholesterol, level). Limit foods high in cholesterol, such as liver and other organ meats, egg yolks, and full-fat dairy products.

Good sources of soluble fiber include oats, certain fruits (such as oranges and pears) and vegetables (such as brussels sprouts and carrots), and dried peas and beans.

Drug Treatment

Even if you begin drug treatment to lower your cholesterol, you will need to continue your treatment with lifestyle changes. This will keep the dose of medicine as low as possible, and lower your risk in other ways as well. There are several types of drugs available for cholesterol lowering, including statins, bile acid sequestrants, nicotinic acid, fibric acids, and cholesterol absorption inhibitors. Your doctor can help decide which type of drug is best for you. The statin drugs are very effective in lowering LDL levels and are safe for most people. Bile acid sequestrants also lower LDL and can be used alone or in combination with statin drugs. Nicotinic acid lowers LDL and triglycerides and raises HDL. Fibric acids lower LDL somewhat but are used mainly to treat high triglyceride and low HDL levels. Cholesterol absorption inhibitors lower LDL and can be used alone or in combination with statin drugs.

Note: Before beginning any diet and exercise regimen, you should speak with your physician to be sure it is right for you. Your physician will also advise you whether you should begin drug treatment to lower your cholesterol level.

Once your LDL goal has been reached, your doctor may prescribe treatment for high triglycerides and/or a low HDL level, if present. The treatment includes losing weight if needed, increasing physical activity, quitting smoking, and possibly taking a drug.

Resources

For more information about lowering cholesterol and lowering your risk for heart disease, write to the NHLBI Health Information Center, P.O. Box 30105, Bethesda, MD, 20824-0105 or call 301-592-8573.

Source: National Heart, Lung, and Blood Institute. (2005). *High blood cholesterol: What you need to know.* Retrieved from http://www.nhlbi.nih.gov/health/public/heart/chol/hbc_what.htm.

Risk Scoring Tables: Estimate of Ten-Year Risk for Coronary Heart Disease

Men
(Framingham Point Scores)*

Age	Points
20–34	−9
35–39	−4
40–44	0
45–49	3
50–54	6
55–59	8
60–64	10
65–69	11
70–74	12
75–79	13

Women
(Framingham Point Scores)*

Age	Points
20–34	−7
35–39	−3
40–44	0
45–49	3
50–54	6
55–59	8
60–64	10
65–69	12
70–74	14
75–79	16

Men

Total Cholesterol	Points				
	Age 20–39	Age 40–49	Age 50–59	Age 60–69	Age 70–79
<160	0	0	0	0	0
160–199	4	3	2	1	0
200–239	7	5	3	1	0
240–279	9	6	4	2	1
≥280	11	8	5	3	1

Women

Total Cholesterol	Points				
	Age 20–39	Age 40–49	Age 50–59	Age 60–69	Age 70–79
<160	0	0	0	0	0
160–199	4	3	2	1	1
200–239	8	6	4	2	1
240–279	11	8	5	3	2
≥280	13	10	7	4	2

Men

	Points				
	Age 20–39	Age 40–49	Age 50–59	Age 60–69	Age 70–79
Nonsmoker	0	0	0	0	0
Smoker	8	5	3	1	1

Women

	Points				
	Age 20–39	Age 40–49	Age 50–59	Age 60–69	Age 70–79
Nonsmoker	0	0	0	0	0
Smoker	9	7	4	2	1

Men

HDL (mg/dl)	Points
≥60	−1
50–59	0
40–49	1
<40	2

Women

HDL (mg/dl)	Points
≥60	−1
50–59	0
40–49	1
<40	2

Men

Systolic BP (mmHg)	If Untreated	If Treated
<120	0	0
120–129	0	1
130–139	1	2
140–159	1	2
≥160	2	5

Women

Systolic BP (mmHg)	If Untreated	If Treated
<120	0	0
120–129	1	3
130–139	2	4
140–159	3	5
≥160	4	6

*The Framingham Heart Study is a long-term ongoing medical study conducted by the National Heart, Lung, and Blood Institute.

Point Total	10-Year Risk (%)
≥<0	<1
0	1
1	1
2	1
3	1
4	1
5	2
6	2
7	3
8	4
9	5
10	6
11	8
12	10
13	12
14	16
15	20
16	25
≥17	≥30

10-year risk _____%

Point Total	10-Year Risk (%)
≥<9	<1
9	1
10	1
11	1
12	1
13	2
14	2
15	3
16	4
17	5
18	6
19	8
20	11
21	14
22	17
23	22
24	27
≥25	≥30

10-year risk _____%

*The Framingham Heart Study is a long-term ongoing medical study conducted by the National Heart, Lung, and Blood Institute.

Chapter 12

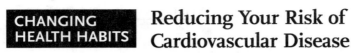

Reducing Your Risk of Cardiovascular Disease

In completing the "Applying What You Have Learned" questions for this chapter in the text-book, you analyzed your lifestyle to determine which modifiable risk factors are raising your probability of developing cardiovascular disease. Then you described how you could mod-ify your behavior to lower your risk of developing cardiovascular disease. Pick one of these behaviors and take the following steps to facilitate change.

Deciding to Change

1. Identify the problem, goal, or question.
2. List the reasons you should make this change and the reasons you should not.

Choices

Reasons to change behaviors (pros):

Points	Reasons
_____	_____
_____	_____
_____	_____
_____ Total	

Reasons not to change behaviors (cons):

Points	Reasons
_____	_____
_____	_____
_____	_____
_____ Total	

3. Draw a conclusion by adding the points in the pros section and then in the cons section. If the point total of the pros section is greater than the total of the cons section, you are probably ready to make a change in your life that reduces your risk of cardiovascular disease. If your cons outweigh your pros, you may not be motivated to make the change now. Study your list of pros and cons carefully, however, before making your final decision. You may decide to change even if your reasons not to change outrank your reasons to change.

Implementing the Change

1. Set a target date to begin the new behavior or reach the goal.
2. Identify and list the factors that will help you reach your goal and those that will stand in the way of reaching your goal.

   Factors that help: _____

   _____

   Factors that hinder: _____

   _____

3. Prepare an action plan for making the change.

   a. Identify alternative methods to reach your goal.

   Alternative 1: _____

   Alternative 2: _____

   Alternative 3: _____

   Alternative 4: _____

   b. Gather information about each method.

   c. Choose the method that fits your situation best.

   d. Consider the factors that can help or hinder your effort to change (see step 2).

4. Change the lifestyle behavior that you have decided to improve by implementing the action plan you developed in step 3.

5. Chart your daily progress toward your goal.

6. Evaluate how effective you were in reaching your goal.

Chapter 13

SELF-ASSESSMENT **What Are Your Cancer Risks?**

Breast or Ovarian Cancer

1. Are you female?   Yes   No
2. Do you have a family history of breast and/or ovarian cancer?   Yes   No
3. Are you over the age of 18?   Yes   No
4. Do you have at least one first-degree relative (mother, sister, or daughter) with breast or ovarian cancer?   Yes   No

If you answered yes to all of these questions, you may be at increased risk of developing breast or ovarian cancer.

Prostate Cancer

1. Are you male?   Yes   No
2. Are you African American?   Yes   No
3. Do you have a family history of prostate cancer?   Yes   No
4. Do you have one first-degree relative (father, brother, or son) with prostate cancer?   Yes   No
5. Was your relative diagnosed at a young age?   Yes   No

If you answered yes to most of these questions, or if you are an African American male, you may be at increased risk of developing prostate cancer.

Skin Cancer (Melanoma)

1. Do you have one or more first-degree relatives (parent, brother, sister, child) with a history of melanoma?   Yes   No
2. Do you experience severe blistering sunburns (especially at young ages)?   Yes   No
3. Do you sit in the sun with the purpose of getting tan, use tanning lamps, or tanning booths?   Yes   No
4. Do you have red or blond hair and fair skin that freckles or sunburns easily?   Yes   No

If you answered yes to any of these questions, you may be at risk of developing skin cancer (melanoma).

Liver Cancer

1. Have you been diagnosed with hepatitis B virus (HBV) or hepatitis C virus (HCV)?   Yes   No

2. Do you drink large amounts of alcohol?   Yes   No

3. Have you been diagnosed with cirrhosis of the liver (a progressive disorder that leads to scarring of the liver)?   Yes   No

If you answered yes to any of these questions, you may be at risk of developing liver cancer.

Gastrointestinal Cancer

1. Do you or one of your close relatives have a history of colorectal cancer, colon polyps, or other cancers (uterine, stomach, bile duct, urinary tract, or ovarian)?   Yes   No

2. Were you previously treated for colon cancer or polyps?   Yes   No

3. Do you have inflammatory bowel disease, such as ulcerative colitis or Crohn's disease?   Yes   No

4. Have you consumed foods that contain aflatoxins? Aflatoxins are a group of chemicals produced by a mold that can contaminate certain foods, such as peanuts, corn, grains, and seeds, and are carcinogens (cancer-causing agents) for liver cancer.   Yes   No

If you answered yes to one or more of these questions, you may be at risk of developing gastrointestinal cancer.

Chapter 13

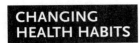 Modifying Behavior to Reduce Cancer Risk

In completing the "Applying What You Have Learned" questions for this chapter in the textbook, you analyzed your lifestyle to determine which modifiable risk factors are raising your probability of developing cancer. Then you described how you could modify your behavior to lower your risk of developing cancer. Pick one of these behavior changes and follow the following steps to facilitate change.

Deciding to Change

1. Identify the problem, goal, or question.

2. List the reasons you should make this change and the reasons you should not.

Choices

Reasons to change behaviors (pros):   Reasons not to change behaviors (cons):

Points   Reasons   *Points   Reasons*

____   _____   ____   _____

____   _____   ____   _____

____   _____   ____   _____

____ Total   ____ Total

3. Draw a conclusion by adding the points in the pros section and then in the cons section. If the point total of the pros section is greater than the total of the cons section, you are probably ready to make a change that reduces your risk of cancer. If your cons outweigh your pros, you may not be motivated to make the change now. Study your list of pros and cons carefully, however, before making your final decision. You may decide to change even if your reasons not to change outrank your reasons to change.

Implementing the Change

1. Set a target date to begin the new behavior or reach the goal.

2. Identify and list the factors that will help you reach your goal and those that will stand in the way of reaching your goal.

   Factors that help: _____

   Factors that hinder: _____

3. Prepare an action plan for making the change.

   a. Identify alternative methods for reaching your goal.

      Alternative 1: _____

      Alternative 2: _____

      Alternative 3: _____

      Alternative 4: _____

   b. Gather information about each method.

   c. Choose the method that fits your particular situation best.

   d. Consider the factors that can help or hinder your effort to change (see step 2).

4. Change the lifestyle behavior that you have decided to improve by implementing the action plan you developed in step 3.
5. Chart your daily progress toward your goal.
6. Evaluate how effective you were in reaching your goal.

Chapter 14

SELF-ASSESSMENT STI Attitude Scale

Directions

••

Please read each statement carefully: STIs are sexually transmitted infections, once called vene-real diseases. Record your first reaction by circling the letter that best describes how much you agree or disagree with the idea.

Use this key:

   SA = Strongly agree; A = Agree; U = Undecided;

   D = Disagree; SD = Strongly disagree.

Remember: STIs means sexually transmitted infections, such as gonorrhea, syphilis, genital herpes, chlamydia, HPV, and AIDS.

1. How one uses his or her sexuality has nothing to do with STIs.

   SA   A   U   D   SD

2. It is easy to use the prevention methods that reduce one's chances of getting an STI.

   SA   A   U   D   SD

3. Responsible sex is one of the best ways of reducing the risk of STIs.

   SA   A   U   D   SD

4. Getting early medical care is the main key to preventing harmful effects of STIs.

   SA   A   U   D   SD

5. Choosing the right sex partner is important in reducing the risk of getting an STI.

   SA   A   U   D   SD

6. A high rate of STIs should be a concern for all people.

   SA   A   U   D   SD

7. People with an STI have a duty to get their sex partners to seek medical care.

   SA   A   U   D   SD

8. The best way to get a sex partner to STI treatment is to take him or her to the doctor with you.

   SA   A   U   D   SD

9. Changing one's sex habits is necessary once the presence of an STI is known.

   SA   A   U   D   SD

10. I would dislike having to follow the medical steps for treating an STI.

    SA   A   U   D   SD

11. If I were sexually active, I would feel uneasy doing things before and after sex to prevent getting an STI.

    SA   A   U   D   SD

12. If I were sexually active, it would be insulting if a sex partner suggested we use a condom to avoid STIs.

    SA   A   U   D   SD

13. I dislike talking about STIs with my peers.

    SA   A   U   D   SD

14. I would be uncertain about going to the doctor unless I was sure I really had an STI.

    SA   A   U   D   SD

15. I would feel that I should take my sex partner with me to a clinic if I thought I had an STI.

    SA   A   U   D   SD

16. It would be embarrassing to discuss STIs with one's partner if one were sexually active.

    SA   A   U   D   SD

17. If I were to have sex, the chance of getting an STI makes me uneasy about having sex with more than one person.

    SA   A   U   D   SD

18. I like the idea of sexual abstinence (not having sex) as the best way of avoiding STIs.

    SA   A   U   D   SD

19. If I had an STI, I would cooperate with public health persons to find the sources of the STI.

    SA   A   U   D   SD

20. If I had an STI, I would avoid exposing others while I was being treated.

    SA   A   U   D   SD

21. I would have regular STI checkups if I were having sex with more than one partner.

    SA   A   U   D   SD

22. I intend to look for STI signs before deciding to have sex with anyone.

    SA   A   U   D   SD

23. I will limit my sex activity to just one partner because of the chances I might get an STI.

    SA   A   U   D   SD

24. I will avoid sex contact anytime I think there is even a slight chance of getting an STI.

    SA   A   U   D   SD

25. The chance of getting an STI would not stop me from having sex.

    SA   A   U   D   SD

26. If I had a chance, I would support community efforts toward controlling STIs.

    SA   A   U   D   SD

27. I would be willing to work with others to make people aware of STI problems in my town.

    SA   A   U   D   SD

Scoring   Calculate total points for each subscale and total scale, using the point values below.

   For items 1, 10–14, 16, 25: Strongly agree = 5 points; Agree = 4 points; Undecided = 3 points; Disagree = 2 points; and Strongly disagree = 1 point.

   For items 2–9, 15, 17–24, 26, 27: Strongly agree = 1 point; Agree = 2 points; Undecided = 3 points; Disagree = 4 points; and Strongly disagree = 5 points.

   Total scale: items 1–27

   Belief subscale: items 1–9

   Feeling subscale: items 10–18

   Intention to act subscale: items 19–27

Interpretation

High score predisposes one toward high-risk STI behavior. Low score predisposes one toward low-risk STI behavior.

Yarber, Torabi, and Veenker (1989) developed the STI Attitudes Scale by administering three experimental forms of 45 items each. Respondents were 2,980 students in six secondary school districts in the Midwest and East. Based on statistical analysis, the scale was reduced to the final 27 items. Reliability coefficients for the entire scale and the three subscales ranged from 0.48 to 0.73. The developers reported evidence of construct validity in that the scale was sensitive to positive attitude changes resulting from STI education.

Chapter 14

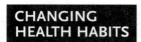 Reducing Your Risk of Contracting an STI

In completing the "Applying What You Have Learned" questions for this chapter in the textbook, you analyzed your risk for contracting STIs. Then you determined what you could do to lower your risk of contracting a sexually transmitted infection. Pick one of these behavior changes and take the following steps to facilitate change.

Deciding to Change

1. Identify the problem, goal, or question.
2. List the reasons you should make this change and the reasons you should not.

Choices

Reasons to change behaviors (pros):		Reasons not to change behaviors (cons):	
Points	*Reasons*	*Points*	*Reasons*
____	_____	____	_____
____	_____	____	_____
____	_____	____	_____
____ Total		____ Total	

3. Draw a conclusion by adding the points in the pros section and then in the cons section. If the point total of the pros section is greater than the total of the cons section, you are probably ready to make a change that reduces your risk of contracting an STI. If your cons outweigh your pros, you may not be motivated to make the change now. Study your list of pros and cons carefully, however, before making your final decision. You may decide to change even if your reasons not to change outrank your reasons to change.

Implementing the Change

1. Set a target date to begin the new behavior or reach the goal.
2. Identify and list the factors that will help you reach your goal and those that will stand in the way of reaching your goal.

   Factors that help: _____

   Factors that hinder: _____

3. Prepare an action plan for making the change.

   a. Identify alternative methods to reach your goal.

   Alternative 1: _____

   Alternative 2: _____

   Alternative 3: _____

   Alternative 4: _____

   b. Gather information about each method.

   c. Choose the method that fits your particular situation best.

   d. Consider the factors that can help or hinder your effort to change (see step 2).

4. Change the lifestyle behavior that you have decided to improve by implementing the action plan you developed in step 3.

5. Chart your daily progress toward your goal.

6. Evaluate how effective you were in reaching your goal.

Chapter 15

SELF-ASSESSMENT **Preparing for Aging and Death**

Answer the following questions. Depending on your situation, some of the questions may not apply.

1. Are you doing anything to increase your chances of living a long and healthy life? ___ Yes ___ No
   If you answered yes, discuss the steps you are taking to live a long and healthy life.

2. How do you want to spend your retirement years?
   Are you doing anything to prepare for retirement? ___ Yes ___ No
   If you answered yes, what actions are you taking to prepare for retirement?

3. How do you feel about elderly people?
   Do you think they are "over the hill" and should be "put out to pasture?" ___ Yes ___ No
   Why do you feel this way about older adults?

4. Do you worry about growing old? ___ Yes ___ No
   If you do, what worries you about aging?

5. Have you prepared a will and a living will or durable power of attorney? ___ Yes ___ No
   If yes, have you informed your family about these documents?
   Have you selected a guardian for your children? ___ Yes ___ No
   Have you discussed guardianship with this individual? ___ Yes ___ No

6. Have you thought about your funeral? ___ Yes ___ No
   If you have thought about your funeral, what kind of funeral would you want?
   Do you want to be buried or cremated?
   Have you discussed your wishes with your family? ___ Yes ___ No
   Have you made funeral prearrangements? ___ Yes ___ No

7. Have you considered donating your body or your tissues or organs after your death? ___ Yes ___ No
   If you want to donate your body, tissues, or organs, have you made any preparations and informed relatives? Do you carry a card in your wallet that identifies you as a donor? ___ Yes ___ No

8. If you were told that you have a terminal disease and have only 6 months to live, how would you spend these last months of your life?

9. Have you written your obituary? ___ Yes ___ No
   What would you like people to remember most about you?
   Examine your responses to these questions; there are no correct answers.

Chapter 15

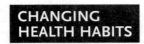

Can Changing a Health Habit Extend Your Life?

Do you have a habit, such as cigarette smoking, that increases your chances of dying prematurely? Which habit? The "Deciding to Change" section of the Changing Health Habits worksheet can help you determine whether you are ready to change this habit. If you decide to change, use the "Implementing the Change" section of the worksheet to help you make the necessary lifestyle changes.

Deciding to Change

1. Identify the problem, goal, or question.
2. List the reasons you should make this change and the reasons you should not.

Choices

Reasons to change
the unhealthy habit (pros):
Points   *Reasons*

_____   _____

_____   _____

_____   _____

_____ Total

Reasons not to change
the unhealthy habit (cons):
Points   *Reasons*

_____   _____

_____   _____

_____   _____

_____ Total

3. Draw a conclusion by adding the points in the pros section and then in the cons section. If the point total of the pros section is greater than the total of the cons section, you are probably ready to make the lifestyle changes necessary to change the unhealthy habit. If your cons outweigh your pros, you may not be motivated to make the change now. Study your list of pros and cons carefully, however, before making your final decision. You may decide to change even if your reasons not to change outrank your reasons to change.

Implementing the Change

1. Set a target date to begin the new behavior or reach the goal.
2. Identify and list the factors that will help you reach your goal and those that will stand in the way of reaching your goal.

   Factors that help: _____

   Factors that hinder: _____

3. Prepare an action plan for making the change.

   a. Identify alternative methods to reach your goal.

   Alternative 1: _____

   Alternative 2: _____

   Alternative 3: _____

   Alternative 4: _____

   b. Gather information about each method.

   c. Choose the method that fits your particular situation best.

   d. Consider the factors that can help or hinder your effort to change (see step 2).

4. Change the lifestyle behavior that you have decided to improve by implementing the action plan you developed in step 3.
5. Chart your daily progress toward your goal.
6. Evaluate how effective you were in reaching your goal.

Chapter 16

SELF-ASSESSMENT 1   Poison Lookout Checklist

The home areas listed below are the most common sites of accidental poisonings. Follow this checklist to learn how to correct situations that may lead to poisonings. If you answer no to any questions, fix the situation quickly. Your goal is to have all your answers be yes.

The Kitchen

	Yes	No
1. Do all harmful products in the cabinets have child-resistant caps? Products like furniture polishes, drain cleaners, and some oven cleaners should have safety packaging to keep little children from accidentally opening the packages.	____	____
2. Are all potentially harmful products in their original containers? There are two dangers if products aren't stored in their original containers. Labels on the original containers often give first aid information if someone should swallow the product. And if products are stored in containers like drinking glasses or pop bottles, someone may think it is food and swallow it.	____	____
3. Are harmful products stored away from food? If harmful products are placed next to food, someone may accidentally get a food and a poison mixed up and swallow the poison.	____	____
4. Have all potentially harmful products been put up high and out of reach of children? The best way to prevent poisoning is making sure that it's impossible to find and get at the poisons. Locking all cabinets that hold dangerous products is the best poison prevention.	____	____

The Bathroom

	Yes	No
1. Did you ever stop to think that medicines could poison if used improperly? Many children are poisoned each year by overdoses of aspirin. If aspirin can poison, just think of how many other poisons might be in your medicine cabinet.	____	____
2. Do your aspirins and other potentially harmful products have child-resistant closures? Aspirins and most prescription drugs come with child-resistant caps. Check to see that yours have them, and that they are properly secured. Check your prescriptions before leaving the pharmacy to make sure the medicines are in child-resistant packaging. These caps have been shown to save the lives of children.	____	____
3. Have you thrown out all out-of-date prescriptions? As medicines get older, the chemicals inside them can change. So what was once a good medicine may now be a dangerous poison. Flush all old drugs down the toilet. Rinse the container well, then discard it.	____	____

	Yes	No

4. Are all medicines in their original containers with the original labels? Prescription medicines may or may not list ingredients. The prescription number on the label will, however, allow rapid identification by the pharmacist of the ingredients should they not be listed. Without the original label and container, you can't be sure of what you're taking. After all, aspirin looks a lot like poisonous roach tablets. ____ ____

5. If your vitamins or vitamin/mineral supplements contain iron, are they in child-resistant packaging? Most people think of vitamins and minerals as foods and, therefore, nontoxic, but a few iron pills can kill a child. ____ ____

The Garage or Storage Area

Did you know that many things in your garage or storage area that can be swallowed are terrible poisons? Death may occur when people swallow such everyday substances as charcoal lighter, paint thinner and remover, antifreeze, and turpentine.

	Yes	No

1. Do all these poisons have child-resistant caps? ____ ____
2. Are they stored in the containers? ____ ____
3. Are the original labels on the containers? ____ ____
4. Have you made sure that no poisons are stored in drinking glasses or pop bottles? ____ ____
5. Are all these harmful products locked up and out of sight and reach? ____ ____

When all your answers are yes, then continue this level of poison protection by making sure that whenever you buy potentially harmful products, they have child-resistant closures and are kept out of sight and reach. Post the number of the Poison Control Center near your telephone.

Source: Consumer Product Safety Commission. CPSC Document 4383.

Chapter 16

SELF-ASSESSMENT 2 **Checklist for the Prevention of Carbon Monoxide Poisoning**

Carbon monoxide is often referred to as CO, which is its chemical symbol. Unlike many gases, CO is odorless, colorless, tasteless, and nonirritating. Red blood cells absorb CO over 200 times more readily than oxygen. As levels of CO in the air rise, this gas replaces oxygen in the bloodstream. As a result, body tissues are damaged and may die of a lack of oxygen. Knowing the major causes of carbon monoxide poisoning and using measures to eliminate them will prevent many needless tragedies.

The following questions relating to various areas in your environment will help you in dealing properly with the unseen, deadly hazard of carbon monoxide. The questions have been divided into sections that may directly apply to your particular situation. You can compare your answers with the correct explanation provided at the end of the list of questions.

Questions

· ·

Draw a circle around your answer.

The Home, Cabin, and Camper

Most questions will apply equally to homeowners, campers, and to those who rent. Renters, however, should refer to the management any questions regarding maintenance.

1. Have you had the fireplace draft and the drafts of other fuel-burning appliances checked by an expert within the past year?	Yes	No
2. Have all gas appliances been checked annually for proper operation?	Yes	No
3. Are all combustion appliances properly vented?	Yes	No
4. Has your chimney vent been checked for defects within the past year?	Yes	No
5. Have you patched any vent pipe with tape, gum, or other substances?	Yes	No
6. Are all horizontal vent pipes to fuel appliances perfectly level?	Yes	No
7. Do you use your gas range or oven for heating?	Yes	No
8. Does the cooling unit of your gas refrigerator give off an odor?	Yes	No
9. Have you ever used a charcoal grill, such as a barbecue grill for cooking within your home, cabin, or camper other than in a vented fireplace?	Yes	No
10. Have you ever brought burning charcoal into your home, cabin or camper for heating purposes?	Yes	No
11. Do you consider portable flameless chemical heaters (catalytic) safe for use in your cabin, camper, or home?	Yes	No
12. Have you ever used a portable gas camp stove in your home, cabin, or camper for heating purposes?	Yes	No

The Auto

13. Have you had a reliable mechanic check the exhaust system of your car within the past year?   Yes   No

14. Do you ever run your auto engine in the garage while the garage door is shut?   Yes   No

15. Do you leave the door closed between your attached garage and your house when you run your car engine?   Yes   No

16. Do you keep your windows slightly open while driving in heavy traffic, although you have an air conditioner?   Yes   No

17. While driving your station wagon, do you lower the tailgate to get a greater flow of air in the car?   Yes   No

Other

18. When you are selecting gas equipment, do you buy only those items that carry the seal of a national testing agency, such as the American Gas Association or the Underwriters' Laboratory?   Yes   No

19. Have you ever converted, or are you about to convert, a fuel burner from one fuel to another without having it done by an expert?   Yes   No

20. As an overnight guest at motels or hotels that have heating units located in the room, do you read operating instructions or ask how such appliances operate?   Yes   No

Correct Answers

....

The Home, Cabin, and Camper

1. *Yes.* A yearly checkup of all fuel-burning venting systems in the home is desirable.
2. *Yes.* A yearly checkup of all combustion appliances is suggested. In many areas, upon request, the gas company will provide this service.
3. *Yes.* All gas appliances must have adequate ventilation so that CO will not accumulate.
4. *Yes.* Chimney vents often become blocked by debris causing a buildup of CO. They should be checked annually.
5. *No.* Often a makeshift patch can lead to an accumulation of CO, and therefore should be avoided.
6. *No.* In-room vent pipes should be on a slight incline as they go toward the exterior. This will reduce leaking of toxic gases in case the joints or pipes are improperly fitted.
7. *No.* Using a gas range for heating can result in the accumulation of CO.
8. *No.* An unusual odor from a gas refrigerator often is the result of defects within the cooling unit. Odorless CO also may be given off.
9. *No.* The use of barbecue grills indoors will quickly result in dangerous levels of CO.
10. *No.* Burning charcoal—whether black, red, gray, or white—gives off CO.
11. *No.* Although catalytic heaters produce heat without flame, combustion is occurring that can cause the production of CO.
12. *No.* Using a gas camp stove for heating the home, cabin, or camper can result in the accumulation of CO.

The Auto

13. *Yes.* Small leaks in the exhaust system of a car can lead to an accumulation of CO in the interior.

14. *No.* CO can rapidly build up while your auto engine is operated in a closed garage. Never run your car in a garage unless the outside door is open to provide ventilation.

15. *Yes.* CO can easily escape from a garage through a connecting door that opens into the house, although the garage door is open. Doors connecting a garage and house should be kept closed when the auto is running.

16. *Yes.* Even with an air conditioner, CO can be drawn into a car while it is being driven slowly in heavy traffic. Therefore, windows should be slightly opened.

17. *No.* If the tailgate is open, be sure to open vents or windows to increase the flow of air in the car. If the tailgate window is open and the other windows or the vents are closed, CO from the exhaust will be drawn into the car.

Other

18. *Yes.* Buy only equipment carrying the seal of a national testing agency; otherwise, one may get poorly designed equipment, which may soon result in the production of CO.

19. *No.* An expert is needed to make proper modifications and to evaluate the venting capabilities of your appliance.

20. *Yes.* Even with adequately designed and properly installed heating equipment, the improper operation of this equipment can result in its malfunctioning and lead to the production of CO. Therefore, be sure you understand the correct way to operate any fuel-burning appliance before using it.

Source: Centers for Disease Control and Prevention. HEW Pub. No.(CDC) 77 8335.

Chapter 16

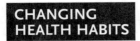 **Can You Reduce Environmental Threats to Your Health?**

In completing the "Applying What You Have Learned" questions for this chapter in the textbook, you analyzed your interactions with the environment to develop a list of environmental threats to your health. Determine ways in which you could change your behavior to remove or reduce these environmental threats. Pick one of these behaviors and use the following steps to facilitate change.

Deciding to Change

1. Identify the problem, goal, or question.
2. List the reasons you should make this change and the reasons you should not.

Choices

Reasons to change behaviors (pros):
Points   Reasons

____ _____
____ _____
____ _____
____ Total

Reasons not to change behaviors (cons):
Points   Reasons

____ _____
____ _____
____ _____
____ Total

3. Draw a conclusion by adding the points in the pros section and then in the cons section. If the point total of the pros section is greater than the total of the cons section, you are probably ready to make a change in your life that reduces environmental risks to your health. If your cons outweigh your pros, you may not be motivated to make the change now. Study your list of pros and cons carefully, however, before making your final decision. You may decide to change even if your reasons not to change outrank your reasons to change.

Implementing the Change

1. Set a target date to begin the new behavior.
2. Identify and list the factors that will help you change this behavior and those that will stand in your way.

Factors that help: _____

Factors that hinder: _____

3. Prepare an action plan for making the change.
   a. Identify alternative methods for reaching your goal.

   Alternative 1: _____
   Alternative 2: _____
   Alternative 3: _____
   Alternative 4: _____

b. Gather information about each method.

c. Choose the method that fits your particular situation best.

d. Consider the factors that can help or hinder your effort to change (see step 2).

4. Change the lifestyle behavior that you have decided to improve by implementing the action plan you developed in step 3.

5. Chart your daily progress toward your goal.

6. Evaluate how effective you were in reaching your goal.